UNIVERSITY LIBRARY
UW-STEVENS POINT

Speech and Language Delay

Third Edition

Speech and Language Delay

A HOME TRAINING PROGRAM

By

R. RAY BATTIN, Ph.D.

*Clinical Psychologist-Audiologist
Director, The Battin Clinic
Houston, Texas
Adjunct Instructor
Department of Otolaryngology
University of Texas School of Medicine
Galveston, Texas*

C. OLAF HAUG, Ph.D.

*Director, Audiology and
Vestibular Department
Medical Center Ear, Nose and
Throat Associates
Clinical Assistant Professor of
Audiology and Speech Pathology
Department of Otolaryngology
Baylor College of Medicine
Houston, Texas*

CRISTINE A. BLAIR, M.A.

*Speech Pathologist
Houston School for
Deaf Children
Houston, Texas*

SUSAN D. MILLER, M.S.

*Speech Pathologist
Outreach Program Coordinator
The Battin Clinic
Houston, Texas*

With a Foreword by

W. LEONARD DRAPER, M.D.

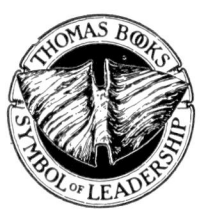

CHARLES C THOMAS · PUBLISHER
Springfield · Illinois · U.S.A.

Published and Distributed Throughout the World by
CHARLES C THOMAS • PUBLISHER
BANNERSTONE HOUSE
301-327 East Lawrence Avenue, Springfield, Illinois, U.S.A.

This book is protected by copyright. No part of it may be reproduced in any manner without written permission from the publisher.

© *1964, 1968, and 1978 by* CHARLES C THOMAS • PUBLISHER
ISBN 0-398-03724-8
Library of Congress Catalog Card Number: 77-21573

First Edition, 1964
Second Edition, 1968
Third Edition, 1978

With THOMAS BOOKS careful attention is given to all details of manufacturing and design. It is the Publisher's desire to present books that are satisfactory as to their physical qualities and artistic possibilities and appropriate for their particular use. THOMAS BOOKS will be true to those laws of quality that assure a good name and good will.

Library of Congress Cataloging in Publication Data

Main entry under title:

Speech and language delay.

    First-2d ed. by R. R. Battin and C. O. Haug.
    Bibliography: p.
    Includes index.
    Appendices (p.   ): I. Children's books and magazines. II. Children's records. III. Parent's books. IV. Organizations. V. Directories and journals.
    1. Speech therapy. I. Battin, R. Ray.
LB3454.B37 1977   371.9'1   77-21573
ISBN 0-398-03724-8

Printed in the United States of America
C-1

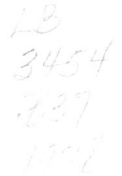

Foreword

A SUCCESSFUL textbook must meet three basic requirements. First, there must be a need for it; second, the information it contains must be presented in a clear, concise fashion so that the reader can easily understand it; and third, the author must have the experience to present the information in an authoritative manner.

As to the need for this book, one needs only to ask the parents of the many thousands of children who have had speech and hearing handicaps to find that such a need has existed for many years. Parents of these children go through three stages in dealing with their children. The first stage is finding out what is wrong with the child; the second stage is acceptance of the fact that there is something amiss; and the third stage is wanting to do something to help the child and looking for the best way to accomplish this end.

The contents of this book are arranged in outline form, making it easy for the parent to find the answer to the specific question that he asks. The book is written in a clear, concise form, in readily digestible points.

Dr. Battin received her doctorate from the University of Florida, was formerly director of the Speech and Hearing Department of Hedgecroft Rehabilitation Hospital, and is a Clinical Instructor at the University of Texas School of Medicine, Galveston, Texas. She is now engaged in the private practice of clinical psychology and audiology. She has had a tremendous amount of experience, particularly with speech-handicapped children. She established the Battin Clinic in 1959 and now serves as the director. The clinic serves children with language-learning disabilities as well as the speech and hearing impared.

Dr. Haug received his doctorate from the University of Wisconsin. He has been engaged in the private practice of hearing and speech pathology for twenty-eight years and was, for ten years, also the director of the Speech and Hearing Clinic at the

University of Texas Medical School. Among his many accomplishments has been the invention of the Pediacoumeter, which has made testing of hearing in the very young child much more feasible than in the past. His infinite patience and exhausting work with the handicapped have resulted in the rehabilitation of many thousands of children in this group. This book then represents a total of many years of accumulated research and work with children who have speech and hearing problems.

As an otolaryngologist who has had both professional and personal experience with these children, I can say that this book will find a most welcome place in the libraries of their parents. The ultimate success or failure of these children to develop to their maximum abilities is dependent to a large degree upon the knowledge and ability of their best teachers—their parents. It is to the development of this parent-teacher that this book is directed.

W. Leonard Draper, M.D.

Preface

THE MATERIAL contained in this book is primarily designed as a tool for parents. The purpose is to set up a workable home program for the development of speech and language in children who are delayed in this area. However, it is the authors' intent that physicians, speech clinicians, and educators should also find this book helpful. It is hoped that it will aid them in working with parents of children with language and speech delay.

The program set forth in the following pages is an outgrowth of an accumulated fifty years of experience in the field of speech, language, and hearing. It grew out of the original authors' need to provide a concrete program which parents of communication-delayed children could follow at home. Many of these families lived in remote areas where professional help was not readily available, and they could only make infrequent trips to urban areas to seek professional guidance.

Definite time allotments for daily therapy were intentionally omitted from the therapy program. It has been our experience that when a definite time segment is set up, parents feel compelled to work within these limits, thus failing to meet the individual child's time capacity. Not only will the time allowed per session vary from child to child, but also from day to day for a single child. It is better to have frequent and short therapy periods rather than one long period. As a general rule, we have found that periods of ten to fifteen minutes twice daily are the most rewarding at first. However, the parent must always be cognizant of environmental and physical pressures of the moment, as well as of daily changes in attention span. She must watch for signs of fatigue, loss of interest, overstimulation, or physical discomfort and should terminate the therapy period or change activities whenever these factors appear. If, however, the child is working well, keenly interested and attentive, the therapy period should be allowed to continue. In other words, the parent working with the child must be flexible enough to fit into the child's working pattern *and not* force the child into another pattern.

Considerable growth has occurred in the knowledge and understanding of speech and language delay and its effect on later learning skills since the publication of the first edition of this book. There are more and improved therapeutic materials available and there is a greater understanding of cause as well as of remediation techniques.

In order to incorporate this material, the original authors asked Ms. Cristine Blair and Ms. Susan Miller to assist us in this revision. Both Ms. Blair and Ms. Miller are outstanding clinicians who have worked extensively with young children having delayed speech and language development. Both hold the certification of Clinical Competency from the American Speech and Hearing Association.

Ms. Blair completed her masters degree in Speech Pathology from the University of Alabama. She has gained experience as a speech clinician at Shadybrook School in Dallas, Texas; the University of Alabama Speech and Hearing Clinic; Center for Developmental and Learning Disorders, Birmingham, Alabama; and as a speech pathologist and teacher of the Multisensory Handicapped at the Arlington Developmental Center, Arlington, Tennessee. Ms. Blair moved to Houston in April, 1976 where she worked with language-learning disabled children at the Battin Clinic. In October, 1977 she joined the staff at the Houston School for Deaf Children where she provides speech and language therapy for the hearing impaired.

Ms. Miller completed her masters degree in Speech Pathology at the University of Oklahoma. She has worked both in the public school as well as a clinical setting, having gained experience as a speech clinician for the Greensburg, Pennsylvania Public Schools; the Somerset County Easter Seal Society, Somerset, Pennsylvania; the University of Oklahoma Health Science Center Speech and Hearing Center; and the Children's Memorial Hospital and the Veteran's Administration Hospital, Oklahoma City, Oklahoma. Ms. Miller joined the staff of The Battin Clinic in August of 1975 and became Coordinator of the Clinic's Outreach Program in July of 1976. She is responsible for an extensive speech, language, and hearing screening program for nursery schools and day-care centers in and around Houston. She also coordinates the Title I learning disabilities evaluation and remediation program for the inner city Catholic Schools.

R. Ray Battin
C. Olaf Haug

Acknowledgments

THE AUTHORS are indebted to the many parents who participated in the early development of this home training program. They are also indebted to those parents who read and commented on the manuscript.

Special thanks are due to Mrs. Mary Robinette, Mr. Oliver H. Smith, Jr., and Mr. Robert Kehoe for their assistance in preparing the illustrations used in the text. We are grateful to Mr. Arthur Brock, Speech Pathologist, M.A., who prepared the illustrations for the revision of the text and permitted us to use his two children in the photographs. Further, we express our appreciation to Mrs. David Marek and her son Wade for allowing us to use their photographs.

R.R.B.
C.O.H.
C.A.B.
S.D.M.

Contents

	Page
Foreword	v
Preface	vii
Acknowledgments	xi

Chapter

I.	How Language and Speech Develop	3
II.	Discipline Training for the Child With Speech and Language Delay	13
III.	The Educational Program	20
IV.	Stimulation	24
V.	Motivation	40
VI.	Ear Training	43
VII.	Auditory Perception	52
VIII.	Visual Perception	58
IX.	The Hard-of-Hearing Child	65
X.	Is My Child Ready for First Grade?	77
XI.	The Parent as a Teacher	80

Appendix

I.	Children's Books and Magazines	83
II.	Children's Records	87
III.	Parent's Books	88
IV.	Organizations	89
V.	Directories and Journals	90

Bibliography	92
Author Index	97
Subject Index	99

Speech and Language Delay

Chapter I

How Language and Speech Develop

MANY PARENTS, physicians, and teachers believe that speech is acquired effortlessly, just as basic motor skills are acquired with physical maturation; that is, at about six months of age an infant is expected to crawl; about twelve months of age, he is expected to walk; and somewhere between one year and eighteen months, most people expect their child to begin speaking. Baby's first step is a much-discussed activity, but less attention is focused on baby's first word. Too often parents are not unduly concerned if that first word has not appeared at one year, nor are they looking for causes for the delay if he is not speaking at eighteen months. We forget that, while a child progresses naturally from sitting to crawling, to standing, to walking, whether he is helped or not, speech is a derivative of social heritage. The child does not progress from crying, to babbling, to talking without help. Lenneberg believes the appearance of language is primarily dependent upon the maturational development of states of readiness within the child coupled with the existence of an adequate environment.

Before we go further in discussing the normal development of speech and language, it is important that we understand the meaning of these two terms.

Language is every form of communication in which thoughts and feelings are symbolized (such as writing, speech, signs, facial expression, gesture, pantomime, and art form). *Speech* is one form of language in which spoken symbols (that is, sounds or words) are used to convey thoughts. Speech is the tool of thought and our primary means of communication.

When the newborn infant informs the world of his arrival with a lusty cry, he has, in a way, begun to speak. For the first two or three weeks of his existence, his vocalizations sound the same no matter what the situation. This expression is innate and reflexive and takes place without intent or awareness on the part of the infant. Toward the end of the second or third week, the world begins to take on form. The child begins to see some order out of chaos and lets us know it by a vocal response. While the child's crying is still reflexive and without intent, there is some relation between the situation and the cry. The mother now recognizes from the infant's cry whether he is wet, hungry, or sleepy; and so the infant is using, in a broad sense, a kind of language. The infant is beginning to control his environment through vocalizations since it does not take long for even a very young infant to discover he can get attention from crying. As the child develops the beginnings of expression, he also begins to be aware of the world of sound; thus, the roots of auditory comprehension appear. When he is about four weeks old, he begins to react to sound.

When the child is about eight to twelve weeks old, he begins to be aware of sounds that he is making. The child has suddenly found that making noise is fun, possibly to hear but *mainly* to *feel*. Therefore, when the infant is enjoying himself, he gurgles, coos, and makes the sounds which we associate with vocal play. This is an important stage in the development of speech and language called *babbling*. Babbling is a delight for both the child and the parent. As the child develops an awareness of his own voice, he also listens to the speaking voice of another person.

While in the babbling stage of development, the child will produce more sounds than are used in the English language. In fact, he probably produces all of the sounds contained in all of the languages of the world. There is no definite order for his acquisition of sounds, but the chances are that he will produce vowels before consonants. The "ah" with variations will probably be heard first. The child, when babbling, is unconsciously practicing his articulation; he is learning to manipulate his tongue and to produce sounds which he will need later. In the early stages of babbling, the infant noisily sucks, clucks, and coos to show how contented he is with life. This oral activity is mainly associated with eating and swallowing and with the pleasure he gets from the sense of feel. Gradually, hearing begins to enter into the babbling, and the infant becomes aware of the sounds he is making. His sounds become more refined and begin to reflect the prosodic pattern to which he is exposed.

To differentiate between the early babbling sounds and the sounds which are associated with hearing, we call this later stage *lalling*. Lalling is the repetition of sounds the infant has heard; this stage appears during the third or fourth month of the child's life. All infants, whether they hear normally or not, go through some form of the babbling stage. However, a severely hard-of-hearing or deaf infant will not develop sounds beyond the early babbling stage without help; he soon gives up these early sounds and sinks into his silent world because he cannot stimulate himself through his hearing mechanism.

The early comfort sounds—the clucks, coos, and gurgles—still remain during part of the lalling period. If you listen to a child closely when he is engaged in this new vocal play, you will find that he varies the intensity, loudness, and seriousness with which he makes his repetitive sounds. These are his to enjoy in private, and any interruption may stop the flow. Since he needs this private practice, interruption by an adult during this vocal play is unwise.

As the child passes into his second six-month period, his sounds become more refined, the vowels are clearer and more pronounced. Between seven and eight months, he begins to vocalize single syllables as *da, ka, la* and such bisyllabic sounds as *ma ma* and *da da*. These are not words; they are still just sounds without meaning. At about nine months of age, the child takes two big steps forward: first, he is able to respond to his name and to the all-important phrase *no no*. Second, he is able to imitate sounds presented to him. At last, the parent's role as a parent-teacher becomes more than one of setting the stage for vocal play. The parent can now fully enter into the game, for the child is ready to imitate the sounds in his environment. We call this stage *echolalia*.

At first the child experiments with the sounds he recognizes, those sounds which he himself made during the lalling and babbling stages. Soon he looks to greener fields and, if the mood is right, will attempt any tongue twister placed before him. It is important that the parents enter into his vocal play since, in this manner, they are preparing him for speech.

As the child and his parents play together with sounds, the child will copy not just the sounds but also the rhythm and intonation pattern presented to him. He will question, command, or complain. This is a signal that he will be saying his first word soon.

Before we discuss this first word, let us go back and talk about the child's comprehension (his understanding of language). In the early stages, his world of language involves understanding gestures, facial expressions, emotional tones of the voice, as well as a few simple words. He will understand speech long before he will use it. In fact, throughout his life, his ability to comprehend will exceed his ability to express himself. Comprehension begins when the infant cries and his needs are attended. It is there when a mother coos or makes loving sounds as she tends her infant and as he smiles in answer to her demonstration of love. Comprehension is also there when she scolds him in a rough or cross tone of voice. The child does not understand the words, but he senses something is wrong from the expression on her face, the tone of her voice, her gestures, and her manner in handling him. He learns to assign meaning to certain things in his confused world of sounds and vision. He knows that certain things represent lack of pleasure.

At about nine months, the child learns to respond to *no no*. However, verbal communication should be accompanied by or reinforced with gesture for the first two years. The early commands *no no, lie down, eat some more, etc.* probably are understood more from the accompanying gesture than from the words.

The first words which a child understands probably are *eat, bye bye, bath,* and *ma ma* and *da da*. This understanding is not as adults know it. The child does not associate the word with an activity, object, or person but rather with a state of being. The word is part of the confused world of sight, sound, touch, taste, and feeling.

To help the child understand, if he is two years or under, talking must be limited. Single words or short phrases, repeated over

How Language and Speech Develop

and over again and always associated with the proper activity, should be used. The child should not be pressed to say them but rather to understand their meaning.

If the child is saying single words, the mother should use two words. For example, if the child says *car*, you should repeat, *car go* and if the child says *car go*, repeat, *car go fast*.

Ordinarily the child has many forms of expressive communication in the pre-speech period other than crying. Usually he has a gesture language which he uses very effectively and which leaves no doubt in the parents' minds as to what he is attempting to communicate. Commonly observed gestures during early babyhood include pushing the nipple from the mouth, or allowing the milk to run out of the mouth—both of which indicate that the baby is not hungry. Smiling and holding out the arms indicate that the baby wants to be picked up. Squirming, wiggling, and crying during dressing and bathing show that the baby resents the restrictions to his activities.

Before we discuss the child's acquisition of true speech, let us stress that, while we have discussed speech development in terms of stages, these stages overlap and are not complete within themselves. Echolalia or imitation and even lalling continue long after the child has acquired real words.

The first true words spoken by a child will either be a single syllable *da*, or duplicated syllable *ma ma*. They will ordinarily appear between ten and fourteen months of age; if true words have not occurred before eighteen months, parents should be concerned. Girls, on the average, will acquire words from one to two months earlier than boys. You may ask why we now label these syllables as *true speech* when earlier we described them as lalling or echolalia. The difference is in the child's reaction to the sound or sounds. These syllables only become true speech if the child uses them to designate a specific object. In other words, the child has learned to talk because he has used a word deliberately and purposefully with the intention of exerting a measure of control over his environment.

You may wonder why we have spent so much time discussing

this pre-speech period. It is important that parents have a sound understanding of the foundation for speech. It is important that they know the child receives physical and auditory pleasure from vocal play, that he controls his environment by gesture, and that he will not develop past this pre-speech stage unless the proper motivation, stimulation and opportunity are placed before him. If, however, the proper stage is set—and assuming that hearing is within normal limits, that there is no neuromuscular involvement of the speech mechanism, that there are no severe structural deformities, and that there is no great intellectual deficit or injury to the language centers of the brain— speech should develop at approximately the following rate (Table I).

The six-year-old has a sentence length of five words, and he uses compound-complex sentences. The average vocabulary is from 2,500 to 3,000 words. The average gain in words per year from two to six years of age is approximately 475 words. The ratio of the various parts of speech in children's language based on total words used is practically unchanged between three-and-a-half and nine-and-a-half years of age. You can see, then, why we say the early preschool years are the most critical in the establishment of speech and language.

Remember, speech and language are learned functions. However, a child needs certain basic things in order to learn these functions. These basic requirements must be met in two areas: (1) within himself and (2) within his environment. Those things that the child requires within himself are as follows:

1. Adequate intelligence.
2. Normal hearing.
3. Properly functioning speech mechanism.
4. Average auditory memory and attention span.
5. Freedom from chronic illness.
6. Freedom from brain injury.
7. Good emotional balance.

Those things that the child requires within his environment are as follows:

TABLE I
LANGUAGE AND SPEECH DEVELOPMENT

Age in Years

	6 months	1	1½	2
Language Understanding and Basic Communication	smiles, laughs	understands "no no" inhibition; knows "bye bye" and pat-a-cake	understands very simple verbal instructions accompanied by gesture and intonation; identifies 3 body parts; points to 5 simple pictures; points for wants	identifies 5 body parts; finds 10 pictures; obeys 1 or 2 prepositions
Appearance of Individual Sounds	7 vowels, 5 consonants in babbling	10 vowels, 9 consonants in babbling and echoing	p, b, m, h, w in babbling	
Auditory Memory Imitation and Repetition		lalls; imitates sound; echoes or repeats syllables or some words (may not have meaning)	repeats some words (may not have meaning)	
Numerical Size of Vocabulary		1-2 words	10-20 words	50-250 words
Word Type		nouns	nouns and some verbs	nouns, verbs, and adjectives
Sentence Length			single words	2 words
Description of Vocalization and Communication	smile, cry, grunt, babble, lall, squeal	babbling, lalling, echolalia	leading, pointing, jargon, some words	words, phrases, simple sentences
Purpose of Vocalization and Communication	pleasure reflexive	pleasure	attention getting	meaningful social control; wish requesting
Speech Content and Style				possessive "mine"; poor vocabulary and grammar
Intelligibility (%)			20 to 25%	60-75% poor articulation
Language Behavior			complete thoughts conveyed by one word with intonation, gesture, etc.	

TABLE I (con'd)
LANGUAGE AND SPEECH DEVELOPMENT

	Age in Years			
	2½	3	4	5
Language Understanding and Basic Communication	points to 15 pictures; obeys 2-3 prepositions	points to 25 pictures; names 20 pictures	knows colors; 4-5 prepositions; what familiar animals do	knows most common opposites
Appearance of Individual Sounds	t, d, n, k, g, ng, in words	$y, f, v,$ in words	sh, zh, th in words	s, z, th, r, ch, j in words
Auditory Memory Imitation and Repetition	can repeat 2 digits; can remember 1-2 objects	can repeat 3 digits; gives 4 lines from memory		can count to ten; can count 4 objects; can repeat 4 digits
Numerical Size of Vocabulary	400-500 words	800-1000 words		
Word Type	nouns, verbs, pronoun "I"	pronouns (you, me), plurals, adjectives	past tenses, comparatives	adverbs, future tenses
Sentence Length	3 words	4 words		
Description of Vocalization and Communication		phrases, longer sentences	complex sentences	
Purpose of Vocalization and Communication		social control, wish requesting	experience relating, information seeking	asks permission; gives excuses; questions actions of others
Speech Content and Style		announces action; gives full name; tells sex and happenings	language reasonably good; limited vocabulary; seeks information in questions	knows to say please and thank you; language good; boastful
Intelligibility (%)	vowel production—90%	75-90%	90%; quite a few articulation errors ($l, r, s, z, sh, ch, j, th$)	some distortion in articulation (r, s, blends); intelligibility good
Language Behavior	developmental nonfluency first noticed	happier than at any time since 18 mo; likes to whisper; responds to whisper	nonfluency prominent; full-volumed yell; easily excited; still whispers some; great extremes	has maturity of speech which gives him freedom and pleasure, demand and command; sometimes appears to have a hearing loss

1. Love, acceptance, and security.
2. Healthy intrafamily relationships.
   a. Good husband-wife relationship.
   b. Good parent-child relationship.
   c. Good child-to-child relationship.
3. Allowance for, challenge to, and stimulation of the child to function at this age level.
4. Allowance of the child to function within his capabilities without undue pressure or unreasonably high standards.
5. Discipline which is appropriate and consistent.
6. Sufficient time, opportunity, and encouragement for self-expression.
7. Stimulation with rich language experiences so that the child will have something to talk about.
8. Good speech standards within the family.

Speech disorders range in cause and complexity. The number of individuals with speech disorders is high. Authorities place the incidence as high as 12 to 15 percent for kindergarten to fourth grade, and 5 percent for the total population.

If a child has no form of verbal or nonverbal language expression at eighteen months of age, the parent should be concerned and seek professional help. If the child has no words at twenty-four months, even though there is no apparent cause, the parents should seek professional help. Remember, the readiness period for speech may be passed by the second birthday. We recommend that the parents seek this help from a speech pathologist or clinician, preferably a person who holds the certificate of clinical competency from the American Speech and Hearing Association.

REFERENCES

Battin, R. Ray: The Development of Language. *International Child Welfare Review*. No. 13, April, 1972.

Gesell, A. et al.: *The First Five Years of Life*. New York, Harper, 1940.

Johnson, Kenneth O.: *Directory*. Washington, D.C., American Speech and Hearing Assoc.

Lenneberg, E. H.: The Natural History of Language. In Smith, F. and Miller, G. *The Genesis of Language*. Cambridge; The M.I.T. Pr., 1966.

Lenneberg, E. H.: *Biological Foundation of Language.* New York, Wiley, 1967.
Lewis, M. M.: *How Children Learn to Speak.* London, George C. Harrap Co., Ltd., 1957.
McCarthy, D.: *The Language Development of the Preschool Child.* Institute of Child Welfare Monographs, Sec. No. 4. Minneapolis, U of Minn Pr, 1930.
Olsen, Willard C. and Lewellen, John: *How Children Grow and Develop.* Better Living Booklets. Chicago, Sci Res Assoc, 1953.

Chapter II

Discipline Training for the Child With Speech and Language Delay

FOR OPTIMUM speech and language learning, the child needs the security and emotional stability provided by good discipline in the home. This training also aids in the development of self-control, attention, and cooperation essential for adjustment to formal learning situations.

We recognize that some behavior deviations with communication-delayed children are organically based (such as those with the brain-injured child) and may respond only to medication to calm their behavior or to nothing at all. Nevertheless, it is safe to say that the majority of our behavior problems have a functional basis. Even the organic difficulties almost invariably have functional, overlaid factors which do respond to careful training in the home. Nancy E. Wood[*] in her study of 1,200 language-delayed children, reports, ". . . There is apparently no relationship between the degree of original behavior (distractibility, perseveration, temper tantrums) and the eventual progress this child *may* make in language development. Many children who have been extremely distractible and perseverative, eventually become well organized in social behavior. But this change in behavior appears to be directly related to the establishment of *routine* by the parents *(which includes firm but kind discipline)* and a professionally planned educational program for the child."

The approach to discipline training with the communication-handicapped child is not basically different from that needed for the child with normal speech and hearing. The difference lies only in the greater importance of an organized, intelligent,

---

[*] Wood, Nancy E.: *Language Disorders in Children.* Chicago, National Society for Crippled Children and Adults, Inc., 1959, p. 23.

and consistent program for this child. Discipline is imperative, then, because

1. You often cannot make the child understand an explanation for your request or demand.
2. The child often cannot hear or perceive danger signals; therefore, he must respect and accept restrictions on his activity and place of play.
3. Frustration level from communication failures is already high, and we must keep other frustrations to a minimum.

In short, we cannot afford to make the usual mistakes in developmental training if we are to give our communication-handicapped child the maximum opportunity to learn and if we are to allow him to become a happy, healthy, well-adjusted adult.

Before we can talk intelligently about an adequate program of discipline, we must first know what discipline is. Much confusion exists because many people tend to equate discipline with punishment. They think that *discipline* means what is *done* to a person when he is disturbing to others; actually discipline is a process of training and learning or of making a disciple of a way of life. This training fosters growth and development and leads to usefulness and happiness. Parents must teach by example because children learn by imitation and practice.

Other parents reject discipline because they mistakenly feel that it is all a matter of placing restrictions in the child's path, thus stifling his creative expression and curbing his personality development. These overindulgent parents may unconsciously create behavioral problems as the child attempts to gain the parents' attention. A completely free rein may give the child false ideas of life which he will find increasingly difficult to follow.

Every child needs the *security of limits*. Think for a moment how you would feel if you drove in a large city and there were no traffic laws, no stop lights, or no signs to guide you or the other traffic. It would be a frightening experience—such as a child's life would be without regulations.

Let us now consider a few helpful suggestions for one satisfactory training program in self-discipline.

1. ROUTINE AND RULES. Any child is decidedly more secure

when he knows *what* he is to do at all times. If a home has a regular sequence of daily activity and some definite house-rules of behavior, then bickering, argument, and tensions are reduced. The child is more likely to be physically and emotionally at ease and, therefore, contentedly follows his regime.

2. DO'S AND DON'TS. Reduce do's and don'ts by following this rough rule-of-thumb. Include regulations—
    a. if they are necessary for the child's safety and for the well-being of the rest of the family.
    b. if they are necessary for the protection of the family's property or for the property of others.
    c. if they are necessary for the character building of the child.

If do's and don'ts are necessary *only* for the convenience or comfort of the adult, try to avoid them.

3. REASONABILITY. Don't invariably ask for the undesirable or prohibit the desirable. You've often heard the adult complaint, "Everything I want to do is either unhealthful, immoral, illegal or fattening." How can an adult who is conscious of society's restraints and yet questions them, expect a child to understand the adults' restrictions and taboos without resenting them? If a behavior problem exists, or if you are trying to improve on poor habits of compliance with instructions, try this method:
    a. Start by asking the child to do the things you *know* he *already likes to do* in order to change his negative attitude toward direction.
    b. Next, ask him to do neutral things that are neither particularly pleasant or unpleasant to him.
    c. Finally, work up to the task or directions which have been disagreeable to him.

4. "TUNING IN." Give the child time to listen—time to "tune-in" to your frequency from his rambling thoughts and attention all over the "frequency band." This is particularly important for the child with hearing or language impairment. Notice that the child does just this when he is talking to you. He continues to say, "Daddy," or "Mommy, Mommy," until you tune him in. He rarely wastes his message until he knows he has your atten-

tion. He knows that, unless he uses this method, his message will go unheard no matter how many times he repeats it. This being the case, why should we rattle off a direction (once, twice, or even three times) before the child is tuned-in, expect that it was given attention and perception, and assume that the child is ornery and stubborn if he fails to respond?

5. VERBAL OR VOCAL RESPONSE. Insisting on some response (such as "Yes, Ma'am," even though not intelligible) is useful to the parent as well as to the child. After it has been habitualized, the response clearly indicates to the parent whether or not the instruction was heard or understood. Parents' use of this verbal response also helps enormously here. Noncompliance can then be dealt with firmly, without indecision or concern regarding the fairness of the judgment. The child also has the comfort of knowing that he will have an adequate opportunity to get the instruction before being accused of defiance or disobedience. The particular words used (whether "yes, Ma'am," "yes, Mommy," or a reasonable approximation thereof) are not as important as the fact that *some* response be made.

6. FOLLOWING THROUGH. Immediate follow-up of an ignored important instruction, once you have established that it was heard or received, is essential to promptness in compliance and to the avoidance of "scenes." Do not wait until you are provoked, exasperated, or desperate. This means that you cannot give an important instruction while your attention is diverted elsewhere. By giving the situation your complete attention, you can then take the child *to* the desired task or *away from* the undesired one, should a response not be forthcoming. Remember, you are helping to teach good habits of listening, attending, and promptness; you do not teach these things by scolding or punishment anymore than you teach good listening habits for speech or music by those methods. If you do follow through, the child will know you "mean business," and few warnings will be necessary—save perhaps an occasional preliminary "count down" for the very young ones. Also, you will be able to remain calm and controlled and will be more likely to avoid unrealistic unenforceable threats, as well as apology, guilt, and "loss of face."

7. CONSISTENCY. Perhaps only complete rejection disturbs a child's security more than does inconsistency. If you expect to get consistency in response to direction, you must provide a consistent stimulus and a consistent expectation of performance from day to day. Dennis the Menace, giving the facts of life to Joey in a cartoon, pinpointed the dilemma in which many children find themselves: "Joey, when *you* want to do something scarey, you're a little tiny boy, but when *they* want you to do something scarey, then you're a great big boy." A reward or punishment which is consistent in frequency of occurrence, in kind, and in application is essential. Also essential is a *united front by both parents* on all policy matters. Let the child always know what to expect of you, and expect the best of him in turn. Chances are, he will not only accept even disagreeable direction but will do so willingly in order to win your approval.

8. PRAISE. *Praise more than you punish,* and this means praise of effort as well as performance. Trying hard shows responsibility even though results are not perfect. However, be sure that the praise is sincere; children will quickly sense if it is false.

Praise your child when he tries especially hard to perform a task or acts in a manner you hope that he will repeat. Ginott places major emphasis on descriptive praise. Telling a child that he is *good* is not bad but it is limiting. An example would be if your child brings you a colorful picture of a house, instead of saying "Good work," perhaps you could say "What a pleasure to look at these! The pink and orange are such bright colors." Modify your praise to the language understanding level of your child.

9. BRIBES. Under no circumstances should parents ever resort to bribes—for example, "I will give you this toy if you stop that." The child may repeat the undesirable behavior, hoping that a toy will again be given to him. Bribes backfire and can cause great harm. They suggest the opposite behavior, encourage deals, and promote the placing of a price tag on being good and responsible.

10. PUNISHMENT. The kind of punishment is not as important as the fact that it should be individualized, appropriate, con-

sistent, calmly and objectively administered, and not humiliating. Be firm but friendly, and do not be afraid of losing the love of your child when punishment becomes necessary. However, do not continue punishing for the same repeated offense. Recognize that a reason usually exists for most repeated, socially unacceptable behavior, just as a cause is present for a physical disorder. Do not look to innate wickedness, stubbornness or immediately assume mismanagement or oversolicitation on the part of your mate or other family members. Look rather to the child's fatigue or basic needs such as food, drink, or elimination. Look to his lack of perception of what has been said to him and to his lack of understanding of what you expect of him. Consider his feelings of jealousy and his failure to get socially acceptable attention.

11. AVOID PERFECTION. Give the child a chance to experiment in new situations. He will learn better from his mistakes and have more self-confidence as a result of your faith in him. Do not be afraid to admit that even you sometimes make mistakes.

12. TRUST AND CONFIDENCE. Show your child that you have faith in him by the responsibility you give him. Expect him to perform and he will. *Believe* the best and you are much more likely to *get* the best.

13. LOVE. Don't be afraid of losing his love by direction, restraint, or punishment. A child *can* understand that it is *because* you love him that discipline and direction are necessary. Proper discipline can actually increase a child's respect and love for the parent. On the other hand, don't be afraid of spoiling him with kindness, affection, and consideration. It is not love, but inconsistency and indecision, that spoils a child.

14. EXAMPLE. Good behavior, like most desirable habits you hope for and work toward in your child, is *caught* better than *taught*. This would be especially true of the child handicapped in hearing or language understanding. You can moralize until you are hoarse, but it doesn't mean much unless the example of conduct you provide is the one you want him to follow.

15. AUTONOMY. Letting a child develop autonomy is not easy for most parents. It is natural to want to hold on, protect, ad-

vise, or control. All parents want to be needed and important to their offspring. Giving autonomy can be seen as actually giving love to your child. Isn't it more loving to let him use his own power to master buttoning his shirt? Providing a helpful guiding hand with gentle encouragement will let him realize his own ability and thus improve his positive feelings about himself.

16. INDIVIDUALITY. A child's feelings, experiences, environments, physical characteristics, and perceptions of others' opinions all contribute to his uniqueness. A child can learn to cope with frustrations, failures, and disappointments, if he has a positive and realistic self-image. This image need not be compared to a brother's or sister's skills or be structured according to your expectations.

REFERENCES

Baumrind, Diana: Parental control and parental love. *Children, 12*:230-234, 1965.
DuBois, F. S.: The security of discipline. *Ment Hyg,* 36:353-372, 1952.
Faber, Adele and Mazlish, Elaine: *Liberated Parents, Liberated Children.* New York, G & D, 1974.
Foster, Constance J.: *Developing Responsibilities in Children.* Better Living Booklets. Chicago, Sci Res Assoc, 1953.
Ginott, Haim G.: *Between Parent and Child.* New York, Macmillan, 1965.
Kratoville, Betty Lou and Schweich, Peter (Eds.): *Hyperactivity: A Meeting of the Minds.* New York, Parent Pr, 1977.
Krug, Othelda I. and Beck, Helen L., M.D.: *A Guide to Better Discipline.* Better Living Booklets. Chicago, Sci Res Assoc, 1954.
Noshpitz, Joseph D.: Can you say "no" to your child? *Children's House,* Nov-Dec, 1966, pp. 6-9.

Chapter III

The Educational Program

LANGUAGE-RETARDED children need a concentrated therapy program which surrounds them with language stimuli, makes them aware of the need for verbal communication, and develops their powers of attention, concentration, auditory memory, and imitation. These needs lead us to four basic requirements of a language-building program: (1) stimulation, (2) motivation, (3) ear training, and (4) increasing auditory and visual memory and retention. In many instances, these therapy needs can best be met by the parent because he is better able to fit the training program to the child's attention span and working period. In addition, there is greater opportunity for carry-over since the child is working within a familiar environment which permits greater identification and restimulation.

Before starting work with the child, it is important that parents set up some goals for themselves. These goals should be—

1. Acquire patience.
2. Remember to treat your child as a *child* and to work at his level of comprehension.
3. Provide the child with successful experiences and set goals which are within his reach.

The tasks which are placed before the child must be of such a nature that they are not overstimulating, overfatiguing, or of such difficulty that he is unable to cope with them. This is particularly true for those children who have suffered brain injury, are mentally retarded, or have emotional problems. These children may show signs of overfatigue, overstimulation, or inability to cope with the situation through compulsively laughing in a defensive manner. Excessive crying, screaming, or withdrawal may also be danger signals.

The child who has a short attention span and who is easily distracted tends to respond indiscriminately because he is unable to separate "self" from his environment and to select stimuli which are meaningful and appropriate to the situation. This results in confusion and inconsistency of behavior. Therefore, it is recommended that a certain place be assigned for working with the child. The place should be uncluttered, without loud colors, pictures, and objects in view. If the child has a room of his own, it is advisable to have a small desk or table in this room where he can work. The room must be simple with a quiet solid color for walls and drapes. Toys should be kept out of sight. The child should be given only one toy at a time to play with until he is able to play constructively with more than one toy and does not merely shuffle them around.

Just as the approach to discipline training with the communication-handicapped child is basically the same as that with the normal child, so the basic approach to speech and language development is the same.

The speech environment which surrounds the child is the main source of stimulation and motivation for speech. Specific training for any child should be *built* upon a good speech environment rather than *substituted* for it. The following do's and don'ts are fundamental to a good speech and language environment; they should serve as a foundation to your training program.

Do's

1. If you have an infant or very young child, you should coo, babble, and gurgle at and with him. In other words, play vocally with your child.
2. Talk, talk, talk with your child about everyday happenings and things. Utilize your daily trips to the grocery store, cleaners, post office, etc. to expand his language experiences.
3. Listen to what he has to say, and listen attentively with active interest.
4. Read to your child and look at pictures together in magazines, books, etc.
5. Play good children's records for your child.

6. Encourage your child to watch television shows, especially *Sesame Street, Electric Company,* and others. Discuss them with your child.
7. Allow your child to express himself creatively in clay, paints, and imaginative play.
8. Play and work with your child at his level.
9. Use simple, clear, precise language when telling something or giving instructions or directions.
10. Set a good example by watching how you make your sounds, pronounce your words, and form your sentences.
11. Be familiar with the steps in language development so that you can seek professional guidance when signs of speech or language delay occur.

Don'ts

1. Do not interrupt your child while he is talking by telling him to slow down, start over, say the word over, or think before he speaks.
2. Do not give your child only perfunctory attention while he is telling you something—by not stopping what you are doing or by otherwise indicating your attention is on other things.
3. Do not ignore signs of speech or language delay.
4. Do not provide your child with an overabundance of toys. Rather, stimulate your child to develop his own play material.
5. Do not cloak your instructions, directions, or descriptions in verbal garbage. Rather, use simple, meaningful language.
6. Do not use verbal threats unless you intend to follow through.
7. Do not make verbal promises unless you plan to fulfill them.
8. Do not talk down to your child.
9. Do not use baby talk with your child.
10. Do not overconcern yourself or give time and training effort to the productive elements of correct speech artic-

ulation. Rather, be concerned with giving the child "something to say" by developing language concepts and vocabulary understanding. Leave the formal aspects of this rather complex task of articulation training to the professional speech clinician.
11. Do not forget that speech and language are learned functions and therefore must be taught. You are *the teacher*.
12. Do not let other family members interfere during his therapy time with you.
13. Do not talk negatively about his speech when he is present.

REFERENCES

Anderson, Virgil A.: *Improving the Child's Speech*. New York, Oxford U Pr, 1954.

Myklebust, Helmer: *Auditory Disorders in Children*. New York, Grune, 1954.

Wood, Nancy: *Language Disorders in Children*. Chicago, National Society for Crippled Children and Adults, Inc., 1959.

Chapter IV

Stimulation

STIMULATION OF THE CHILD with language forms is the first requirement for both language comprehension and speech production. It is the basic tool by which communication ability is developed. Parents frequently are guilty of failing to take advantage of language stimulation opportunities. Consider, for instance, the times we go riding in the car or bus with the very young child. How often do we make a simple observation such as "there is a dog" or "look at the man?" Fortunately for most children, language growth is not seriously impaired by this lack of stimulation. However, this definitely is not true of the child with delayed language development. Remember, he needs to hear about the common everyday situations and objects, not the unusual ones.

The child must hear in order to be stimulated by language forms. Normal hearing is essential for the development of speech, language, and auditory processing skills. Research has shown sensory deprivation causes central auditory abnormalities. Auditory sensory deprivation may occur through lack of stimulation in the environment or from a failure to receive, i.e. inability to hear, the stimulation that is present in the environment. Marion Downs* defines the criteria for a handicapping hearing loss as:

1. Hearing level of 15 dB or greater;
2. Indications of serous otitis media in a child under two years of age more than half the time for a period of six months;
3. Fluctuations in hearing levels due to recurrent otitis media, with the hearing worse than 15 dB more than half the time over a six-month period.

Mild hearing loss from ear disease in infancy can cause significant language retardation in children, yet these mild hearing

---

* Downs, Marion P.: Deafness in Childhood. In Bess, Fred. (Ed.): *The International Symposium on Deafness in Children*. June, 1976.

losses frequently go undetected. As a parent, be assertive, insist on regular checks of your child's hearing. If a middle ear disease is present, request a hearing test be made which will provide you with an accurate level of your child's hearing. If the hearing is depressed more than 10 dB, be concerned and seek active treatment of the problem. Of course, prevention of ear disease is best. Ask your pediatrician how you may prevent ear disease in your child, thus avoiding later problems. If your child has a sensorineural hearing loss, amplification is essential for language and speech development.

Parents of speech-handicapped children all too often make the gross error of thinking, "What's the use of talking so much to the child, he doesn't understand anyway." Actually he needs to receive more, not less, stimulation than the average child. The constant chatter of a young mother to her week-old or month-old infant, so essential to his early language awareness, is never limited by reservations as to the amount which is being comprehended. She just talks; that is what parents of language-delayed children must do—talk, talk, talk. Of equal importance is the fact that this stimulation must take the form of talking about simple, commonplace objects and activities encountered every day. This talking must occur at the moment when these objects and acts are in view. While we are in the kitchen, we must talk about things in the kitchen, while on the farm, about objects actually seen there. It is best to stay within a close range, speaking directly to the child so that he can watch your face and not be distracted by other environmental noises. Even the simple act of opening a door or walking up stairs can be used for stimulation. We must talk about these acts as they are being performed. It is only through associating what he sees, feels, and smells with accompanying words he hears, that the child will begin to attach meaning to these verbal symbols. This kind of stimulation requires no extra time but can be incorporated into the daily routine. What is suggested is a detailed running commentary on all the day's activities and a description of the objects which are used in these activities. Instead of sending the child away while you are mixing a cake, place a stool beside your work area and let him sit and watch while you describe, step by step, what you are doing.

It is advisable for these children who have no language to advance through babbling, jargon, and gesture stages of language. They must learn to play with sound before being forced to say a word, since in all children, language comprehension and sound play precede meaningful speech production. Also, through jargon, the child acquires the rhythm and intonation of the language.

Ways to Stimulate Language in the Home

1. Since speech grows out of swallowing, chewing, and sucking, encourage your child to acquire good habits of eating, that is, being able to chew and swallow a proper solid food diet. Keep the feeding period a pleasant experience, and use it as a means of simple sound stimulation.

2. Provide the child with as near normal hearing as possible for as much time as possible during his waking hours. If the child has an identified moderate to severe sensorineural hearing loss, provide him with amplification by having an ear examination from an ear, nose, and throat specialist and a hearing aid evaluation by a qualified audiologist. If your child has recurrent middle ear disease, be assertive with your pediatrician or ear specialist. If the hearing cannot be maintained at normal levels the majority of the time, request a mild hearing aid be prescribed so that your child is not deprived of the proper auditory stimulation which is critical for normal development of central auditory skills.

3. Name all objects with which your child comes into contact. For example, when you give him a glass of milk, say the word *milk* but do not pressure him to repeat the word or to respond in any way. Use this procedure with all objects your child encounters: water, glass, cup, sucker, bread, bed, shoes, socks, etc. As the child begins to associate names with objects, introduce short phrases and sentences, varying the form and word order, using much repetition.

4. As your child's associations grow in his everyday environment, expand his vocabulary by making him a language notebook. If your child has the coordination skills, leaf through

magazines and help him cut out pictures. Set up separate sections in the notebook so that you can group items into the following categories:

Animals	Household items
Body parts	Family members
Clothing	Toys
Foods	Transportation
Furniture	Public places (stores, restaurants)

5. Demonstration, pictures, books, and playing games such as *Follow the leader* and *Red light, green light* can be used to teach basic actions, such as running, hopping, sleeping, eating, jumping, etc.

6. Find opportunities to emphasize different parts of speech, such as pronouns (I, me), possessives (Daddy's car, Mommy's shoe, my turn, your turn), negatives (no candy, not happy), and interrogatives (who, what, where, when, why). A few suggested activities are (1) Hide an object and have the child repeat after you, "Where is it?"; (2) Have the child separate Daddy's clothes from his own clothes; (3) Complete a simple puzzle while specifying *my turn, your turn*.

7. Describe objects so that your child begins to develop concepts of spatial relations, color, and form. Include some or all of the following properties:

Size (big, little)
Shape (circle, square)
Color (blue, red)
Volume (full, empty)
Texture (rough, smooth)
Number (one, two, few, all)
Position (on, in, under)

A child needs experience with these properties before concepts are fully established. Play a game in which he puts big objects in a big box and little objects in a little box. Have the child place a ball under the table, on the chair, in the corner, behind the door, or in front of the television.

Remember that the key to successful language teaching is simplicity and repetition of the same concept in varied situations.

8. Young children love the sound of a friendly voice. They

take particular delight in it if the words they hear are rhythmical or rhyming. Children like the repetition of sounds, and they like to imitate and play with them. To provide the stimulation for this sound play, repeat nursery rhymes to your child constantly. Children also need to hear the old favorite lullabies. Play children's records, encouraging your child to clap his hands and attempt to sing along.

9. Read simple children's books to your child and read the same story over and over again (Fig. 1). It is suggested that you have such books as *Mother Goose, Winnie the Pooh,* Dr. Seuss stories, and Richard Scarry's books. (A recommended reading list may be found in Appendix I.) This reading must not be a forced activity for either the parent or the child. If time does not permit, the child will gain more from talking about everyday activities than forced, unhappy reading sessions.

10. Lotto games, matching picture cards, and simple puzzles are useful activities for teaching language (Fig. 2). Be sure to

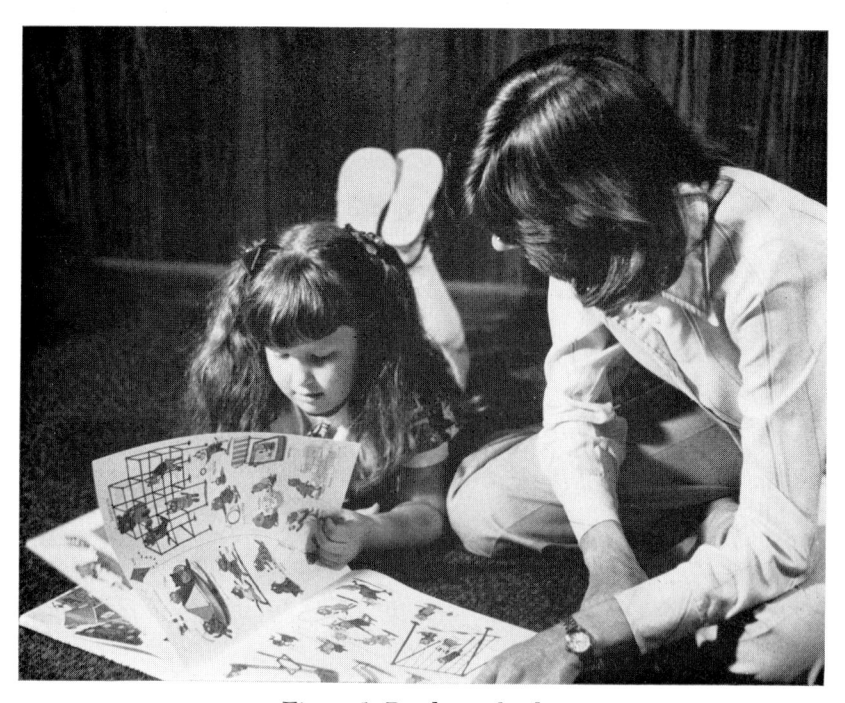

Figure 1. Reading a book.

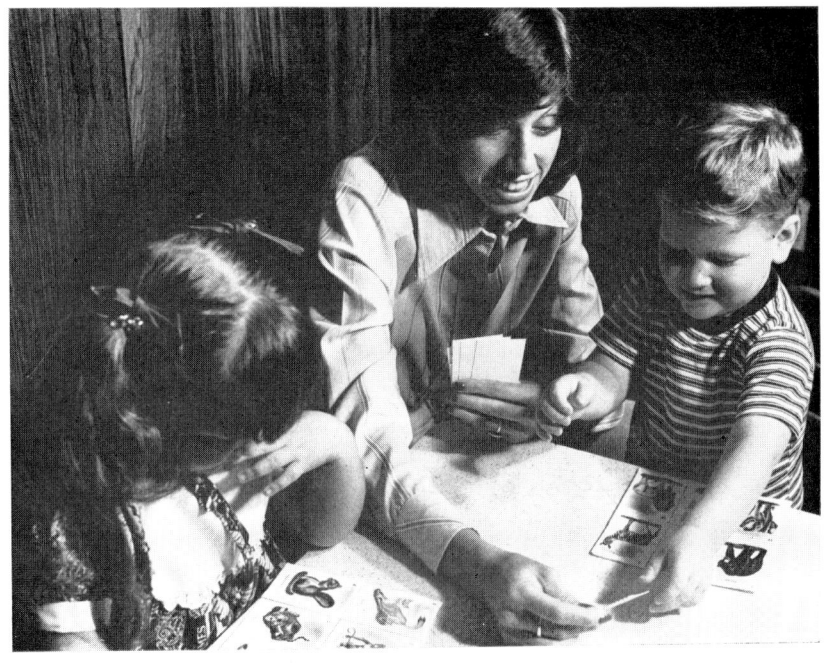

Figure 2. Picture lotto game.

name the cards or puzzle pieces as you hand them to the child. If the puzzle or lotto game depicts a scene, describe it for the child, then later let him do the naming or telling. Accept his words or description, but repeat after him in the correct form. For example, "Yes, Michael, that is a big dog."

11. Purchase or make a flannel board. A flannel board is relatively inexpensive and can be obtained at most teacher supply stores or educational toy stores and some toy sections in department stores. Felt squares in various colors may be purchased from most five-and-ten stores. The flannel board and figures will be useful for many phases of language and speech training and can be used later when your child enters school to teach number concepts.

Cut out simple outline figures from felt, or purchase story figures from educational toy stores or teacher supply stores. Examples of some of the commercially available story figures are "The Three Bears," "The Three Little Pigs," "Red Riding

Hood," and "The Family" (Fig. 3). If you make your own figures (which is less expensive), cut a horse, tree, car, mother, father, girl, boy, dog, baby, and cat as your first group. Make up stories using these figures; keep your language and story simple. For example,

> Almost everybody in the *family* was asleep: Mother, Daddy, Baby, Brother, Sister, and Cat. Dog was outside under the big tree playing. He forgot the family was sleeping and began to bark, "woof-woof, woof-woof." What fun to bark at the moon, "woof-woof, woof-woof." Sister woke up and came downstairs; "sh, sh, sh, sh, Dog," she said. Dog only barked louder, "woof, woof." Brother and Daddy woke up and came outside to see what was making Dog bark. "Sh, sh, sh, Dog," Daddy and Brother said, but Dog only barked louder, "woof, woof, woof." Mother came to the window, "sh, sh, sh, or you'll wake Baby." "Woof-woof," went Dog; "wah-wah," cried Baby. Then Dog went in the house and fell asleep. Brother, Sister, and Daddy went in the house and went to sleep. Mother rocked Baby who did not go to sleep.

As you tell the story, move the figures on the flannel board to

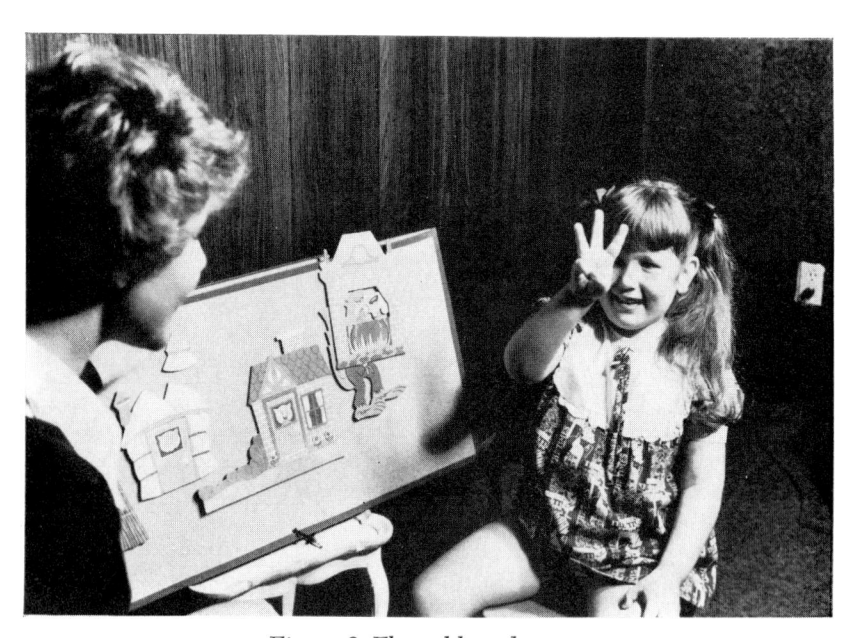

Figure 3. Flannel board story.

act out the story. In this way, you teach language concepts (such as in, on, under, outside, asleep, awake, quiet, and loud).

Build or purchase a series of flannel board figures for language development. Teach previously mentioned vocabulary and expand with more specific items (Fig. 4). Some additional classifications are as follows:

>	Christmas tree with ornaments
>	Easter Bunny with eggs and basket
>	Halloween pumpkins, goblins, witches
>	Thanksgiving turkey, Indians, Pilgrims
>	School items
>	Weather
>	Counting
>	Alphabet letters

12. The flannel board can also be used for teaching form perception.

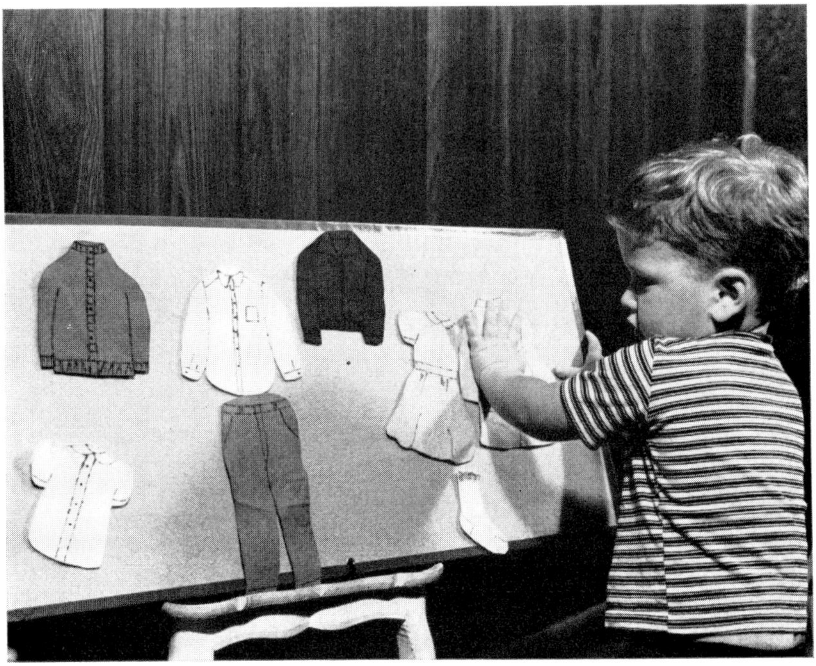

Figure 4. Flannel board clothing.

Cut three circles, three squares, and three triangles from felt. Cut one of the circles in half and the other in fourths. Cut one of the squares in half and the other into four equal squares. Cut one of the triangles in half and the other into four parts (see Fig. 5). You may use different colors for the circles, squares, and triangles, or the whole figures can be one color with the halves in a different color, and so on.

First, use the forms for matching. This will help develop form perception and recognition of the relationship of the part to the whole. Place the circle on the flannel board and hand the child the two halves. The child should then place the two halves on the circle. Next, hand him the four "pies" and have him place them over the two halves. When he is able to do this with

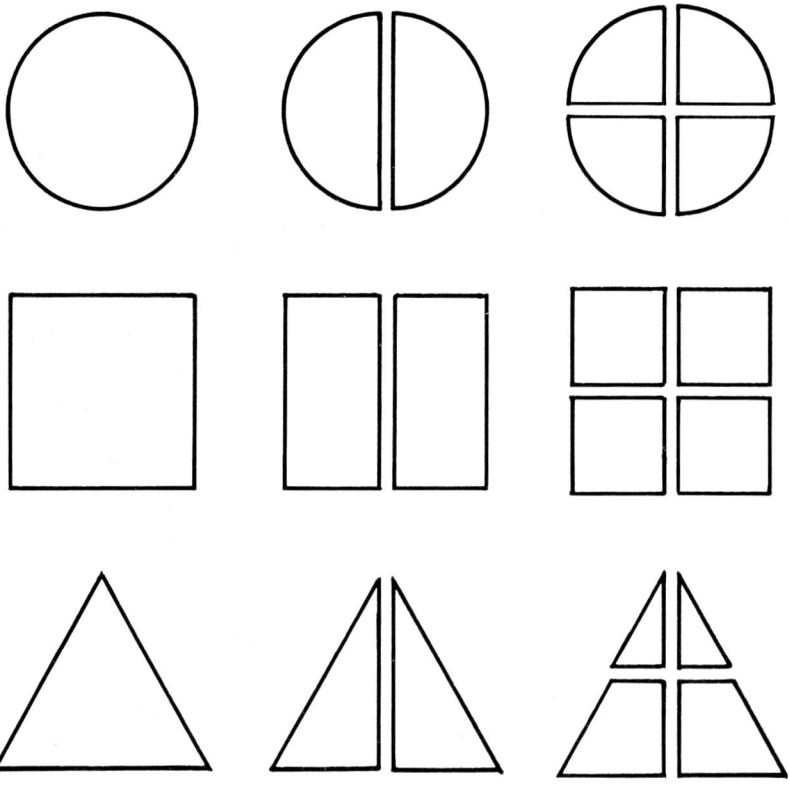

Figure 5. Form-perception figures.

ease, have the child put the halves together beside the whole figure, and the quarters together beside the halves. Work with the square next and then the triangle. Do not move to the square until the child is able to work both steps of the circle without difficulty. When the child is able to put the three forms together with ease, let him paint "felt pictures" with the material. You will need to cut out several small circles for use as eyes, nose, and mouth, along with some strips approximately 3 inches long and ¼ inch wide. Place all the forms, small circles, and strips in a pile; allow the child to "paint" freely. At first, there may be no form to his placement of felt pieces. However, let the child talk with you about his "picture," and praise him for his creation. Gradually, as he plays with the material, he will begin to see relationships between forms, and objects will begin to take shape. Such things as a kite, house and fence, boy, girl, car, and airplane will begin to appear on the flannel board.

13. As your child progresses and matures, he will express an interest in everyday things around him. When he does this, begin to give him such tasks as setting the table, clearing the table, drying the dishes, and making his bed. Always accompany these tasks with verbal instructions even though they need to be pointed out or demonstrated. Accept the fact that the child may appear awkward at first, be patient, let him try, and always compliment him.

14. A dollhouse, furniture, and family figures can be used to allow the child to act out some of his feelings of aggression and hostility toward family members. If the child has some words, the house and its contents can be used to teach language concepts (such as in the house, outside, on the floor, under the table, upstairs, downstairs, etc.) (Fig. 6). Packing a suitcase is a good way to learn and classify clothing items.

15. Hand puppets made from old socks or purchased from a toy store can also be used for sound play and speech stimulation. Finger puppets are fun to make. Dramatize familiar stories or let the child make up his own story. The parent may enter into the story or let the child do it in his own way.

16. A good way to stimulate speech is to have a tea party. Sometimes serve milk and cookies; at other times, have a pretend

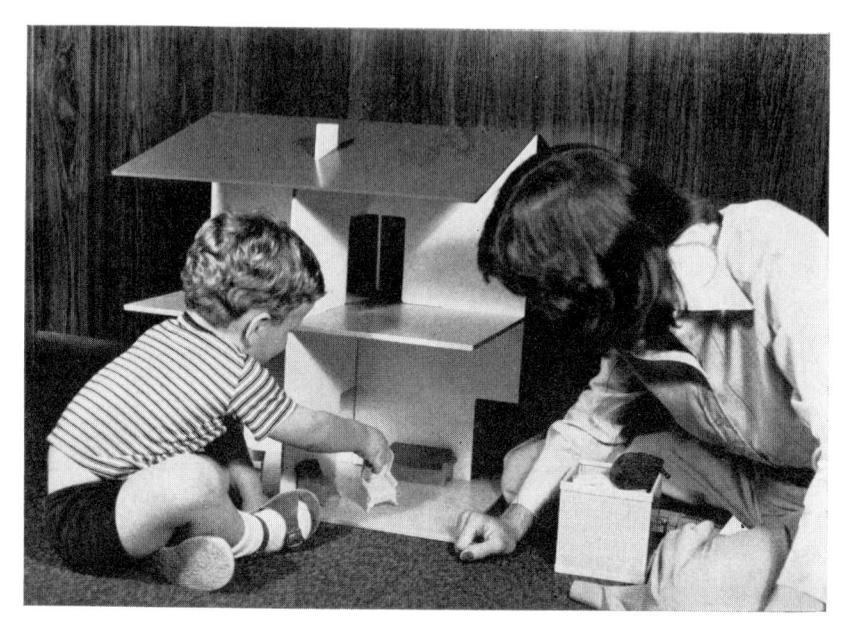

Figure 6. Use of the dollhouse for language stimulation.

party. Encourage sounds by frequent use of "mmm—good" and "more."

17. Working with modeling clay can serve two purposes for your child: (1) it offers a form of expression, and (2) it is a means of releasing tensions and frustrations. It is suggested that you use plastic clay which can be obtained from the dime store. Let the child mold it, pound it, and tear it apart (Fig. 7). Work with the child in molding airplanes, cats, snakes, and other things. Name these things and hand them to him. Do not be alarmed if he "kills them" or pulls them to pieces in an aggressive manner. This is his means of release, and it is a necessary and important step in his development. As his play with the clay is modified, let him trace outlines in the clay with a stylus. This will provide kinesthetic cues which will supplement written language attempts. Here are three different recipes for modeling clay which you can make at home:

1. Blend together 1 cup salt, 1½ cups flour, ½ cup water, 2 tablespoons vegetable oil, and a few drops of food coloring. This

Stimulation 35

blend is nontoxic, and a small child can put the clay into his mouth without harm. Before the child handles it, remember to dust his hands with flour to prevent the dough from sticking.

2. Pour soapflakes into a bowl and stir in a tablespoon of water at a time, until the soap is thick enough to mold.

3. Blend together 1 part salt, 1 part flour, and ½ part water until the mixture is soft and smooth. This should be stored in an airtight container in the refrigerator. Use it up within four days.

18. Painting is another means of expression and of releasing feelings of aggression and frustration. It is suggested that you

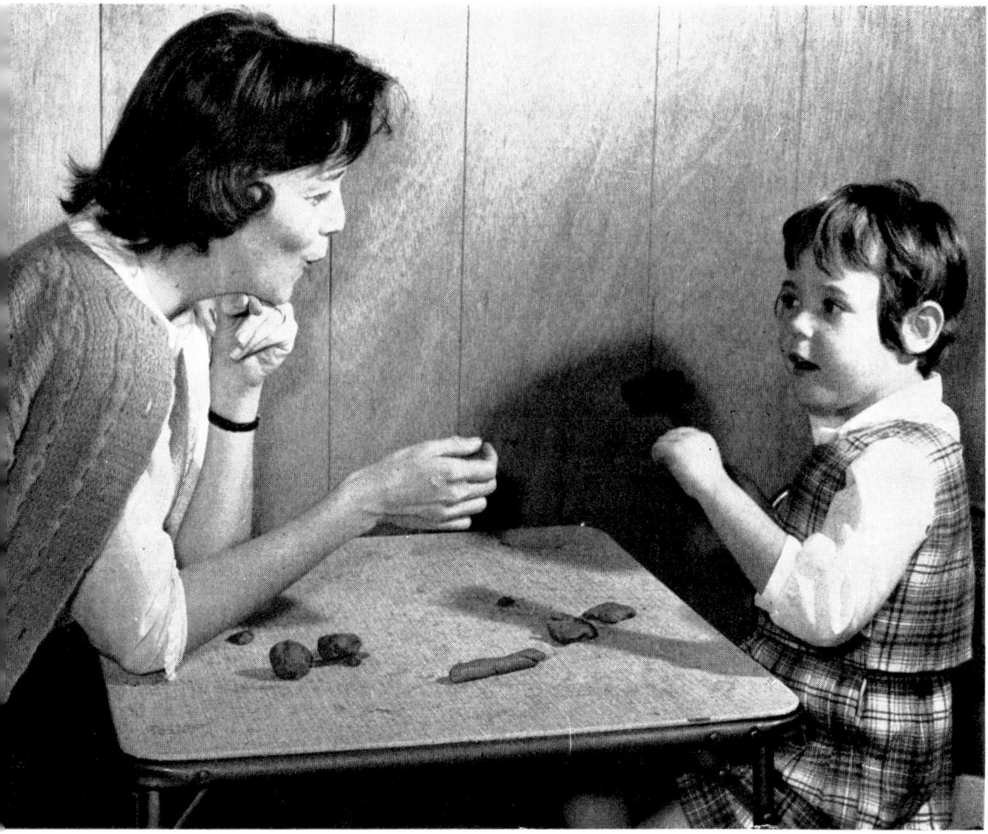

Figure 7. Working with clay. (Courtesy of Ray Covey, *The Houston Post.*)

give your child the opportunity to do both finger painting and brush painting. Finger paint sets can be obtained from any toy store. These sets should include the paints, paper, and a book of instructions. For brush painting, buy tempera paints either in the powder or liquid form. Use a number six paintbrush or one of comparable size. You can also use the ½-inch regular paintbrush found in the hardware store. If your child has difficulty handling the paintbrush or if he is reluctant, at first, to put his hands in the finger paints, mix together tempera powder, liquid starch, and water in empty roll-on deodorant bottles. The child can then paint by rolling the applicator across the paper (Fig. 8). You need to get black (at first this may be the child's favorite color), red, yellow, and blue tempera. You will get purple, green, and orange by mixing the following colors:

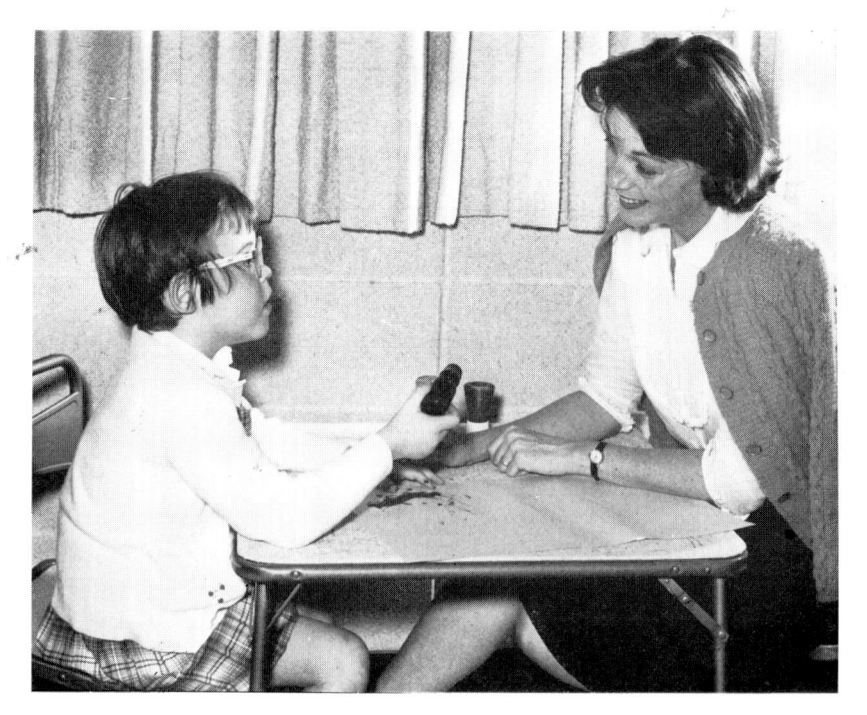

Figure 8. Roll-on painting. (Courtesy of Ray Covey, *The Houston Post.*)

Mix	To Get
yellow and blue	green
red and blue	purple
red and yellow	orange

Newsprint paper, old newspapers, brown or white wrapping paper, and paper bags will serve as paper for painting. You can make a smock for your child to use while painting by removing the sleeves and collar from a man's shirt (Fig. 9). Place the shirt on him so that it buttons down the back. It is best for the child to do the finger painting on the floor. Be sure to have plenty of old newspapers under the paints and under the paper which he is going to use so that you can be relaxed regarding his getting paint on the floor. Remember, this is to be a fun, worthwhile experience for your child. If you are tense or worried about the mess he will make, the child will reflect your feelings. You must display a deep interest in what he is doing. Giving make-be-

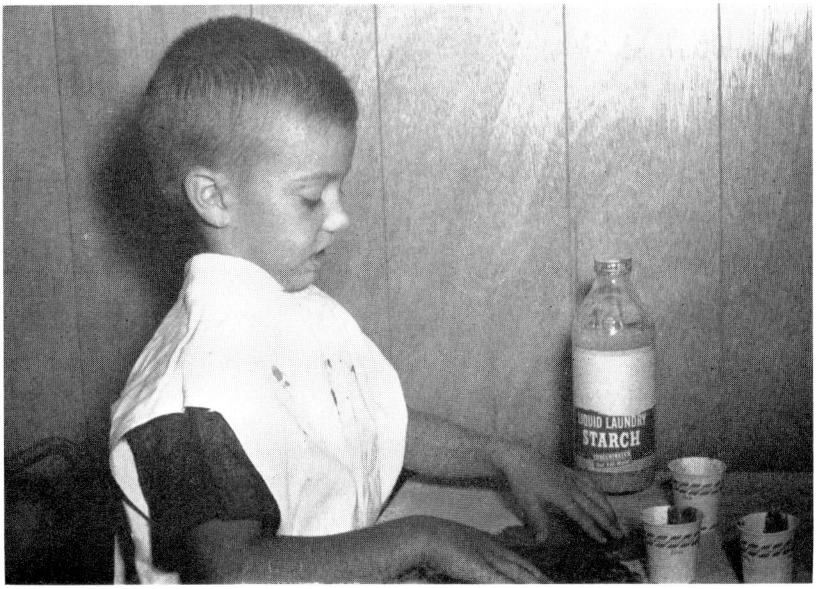

Figure 9. Finger painting.

lieve names to his make-believe shapes may motivate him toward simple sound imitation. The same can be done with the clay.

19. Buy or exchange simple form puzzles with your friends. Be sure they are simple and do not consist of too many pieces. When you present the puzzle to the child, remove each piece in a logical order, naming each part in turn. Do not complete the puzzle for him but offer assistance when he is having difficulty. You might remove only a portion of the puzzle for him to complete. Later, allow him to complete the entire puzzle. Try to help him work it out by himself.

20. Pounding boards, pegboards using colored pegs, block construction, and toys such as Legos™, Tinker Toys™, Lite Brite™, etc. help develop eye-hand coordination, as well as color sense (Fig. 10). They also aid in developing a sense of rhythm, noise imitation, and serial-number stimulation. Remember, the toys must be simple in design. A pegboard can be used in tracing and copying shapes and objects. Name a common object (chair) and

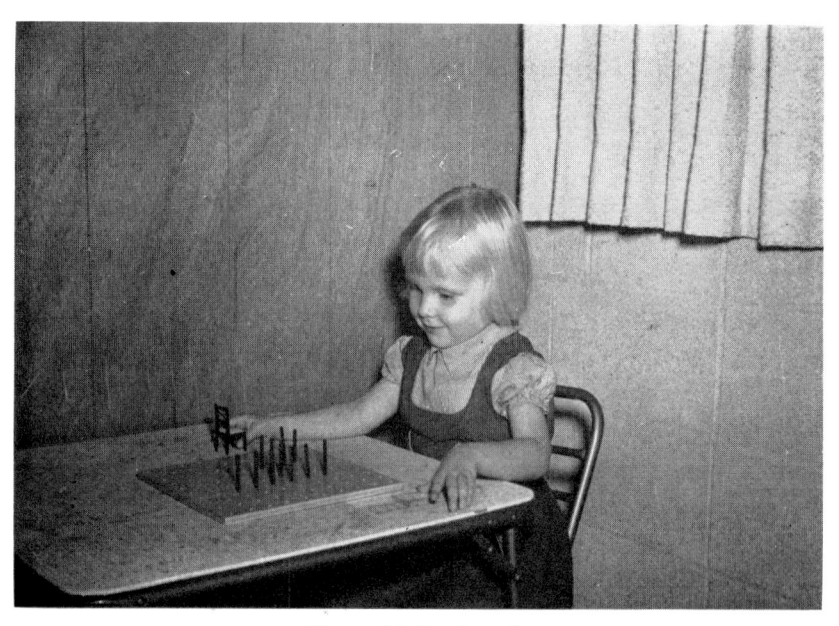

Figure 10. Pegboard.

have the child attempt to trace the object first with his finger, later with pegs. If necessary provide a model for him to copy.

21. Provide your child with old clothes and shoes so that he can play *grown-up*. This *pretend play* is important in the development of *inner* language and imagination. However, you should be cautious and not present these articles too soon in your child's development. Wait until he has acquired sufficient language to enter into imaginative play. You will see this develop in his work with clay, paints, pictures, and small toys.

22. It is important that you talk to your child about everyday activities as they are being viewed. Do not set aside a separate time for this; rather, discuss the situations as they occur.

23. Set up a routine for yourself and adhere to it. Remember, the child learns from everything he experiences; therefore, a calm, harmonious home environment is important.

24. Do not feel that the child must be looking at you or closely attending to your speech in order for that speech to be effective in developing communication. It is enough that he is in the same room, however absorbed he may be in other activities. Keep talking!

REFERENCES

Collins, Norman et al.: *Teach Your Child To Talk, A Parent Handbook.* New York, CEBCO Standard Publishing, 1975.

Downs, Marion P.: Deafness in Childhood. In Bess, Fred (Ed.), *The International Symposium on Deafness in Children.* June, 1976.

Downs, Marion P.: Hearing Loss, Definition, Epidemiology and Prevention. *Public Health Review.* Vol. IV, July-Dec, pp. 225-380, 1975.

Lewis, Neil: Otitis Media and Linguistic Incompetence. *Archives of Otolaryngology,* Vol. 102, July, pp. 387-390, 1976.

Northern J. L. and Downs, M. P.: *Hearing in Children.* Baltimore, Williams and Wilkins, 1974.

Chapter V

Motivation

THE SECOND BASIC REQUIREMENT for developing a child's interest in and need for communication is motivation. Speech is a learned function; as such, it requires considerable effort. Two of the main reasons that children have for putting forth this effort are (1) to get satisfaction of their wants with greater speed or less expenditure of energy than by other means, and (2) to get praise and reward as a result of pleasing their parents. The appeals used by the parents should be immediate, concrete, and of a positive nature. For example, you would not use, "Don't you want to talk like Mommy or Daddy when you grow up?" as a means of motivation.

Also you would not hold an item such as a pencil or a piece of candy in front of the child until the child has said the word. This is not motivation but, rather, a situation which creates frustration. When you hold the child's desired object out of his reach but in his view (as one does in making a dog do tricks), the child knows that you comprehend his request. He also knows that you are only asking him to drill and perform. This is usually irritating and frustrating to the child delayed in language. It is not the proper motivation to which we refer. However, if you let him know that you do not understand what he wants, he knows he is not getting through to you, and he is then motivated to continue his attempts to communicate.

If you really don't understand him, use the same procedure of making him struggle momentarily to make his wants known. Only then should you resort to trial-and-error offering of possible choices or to having the child lead you to the object in question.

Ways to Motivate Speech in the Home

1. If gesture is the only form of language, it should be accepted but reinforced by the parent verbalizing the needs. As soon as vocalization appears, insist that it accompany the gesture.

Motivation

In other words, don't accept less than the best your child is able to produce. In order that a child appreciate the necessity of verbalizing his wants, he must have difficulty in his gratification by other means. Thus, even though you know exactly what he wants by other situation cues, you must pretend that you do not understand him when no verbalizations or vocalizations are attempted. Make him struggle for a moment; if the response is not forthcoming after several trials, fulfill his request. Do not be discouraged by reactions of shrugging his shoulders, getting the desired object himself, and temper tantrums. Perseverance on the part of the parent is necessary.

2. Do not anticipate his needs so that speech is unnecessary.

3. Do not force your child to complete a speech task which at the moment he is unwilling to do.

4. Do not resort to a trial-and-error form of search for an understanding of his wants until he has struggled to convey meaning through language. If you must resort to trial and error, give the child several alternatives from which to choose. Invent alternative choices when asking the child his particular wish in any given situation to prevent nodding, shaking the head, or grunting (for example, "Would you rather have a popsicle or ice cream cone?" "Would you like to go to the zoo, or go to the show?").

5. Do not be moved by your feelings of sympathy to oversolicitation in your demands for speech.

6. Do not let time pressures prompt you to accept partial effort rather than taking the time to demand maximum effort.

7. Speech situations, if they are to be of maximum benefit for the child, should be pleasant experiences.

8. Don't reward bad behavior or lack of speech by dwelling on them. Many times parents make an issue of an undesired behavior pattern; this, in turn, motivates the child to continue this behavior in order to perpetuate the attention. If the child feels the need for attention, he will seek it even though it would seem to be unpleasant. Constant yelling at a child to stop an undesirable pattern or demanding a performance is *not* motivation. We do not mean to imply that permissiveness is the answer, but rather a sound discipline program should be followed such as discussed in Chapter II.

9. Just like gesture, facial expression is a part of communication. It conveys meanings (such as approval, disapproval, frustration, worry and anxiety, acceptance, pleasure and displeasure). Thus, if the expressions are pleasant, they can encourage and motivate; if they are unpleasant, they can discourage or inhibit the child in his speech and listening attempts. One must realize that the child can derive attention from negative as well as positive comments.

It is difficult to separate motivation and stimulation. The important thing to remember in the initial stages of language training is that the child is like a sponge which absorbs a tremendous amount before it begins to leak. You must concentrate on *giving* language to him before you expect him to perform by giving speech to you.

In order to give this speech to you, he must be inspired, must feel a need, and must feel there is sufficient reward. In other words, the child must *want* to put forth the effort required to complete the speech act.

REFERENCES

Sheer, D. E.: Is there a common factor in learning for brain injured children? *Except Child, 21*:10-14, 1954.

Van Riper, Charles: *Teaching Your Child to Talk.* New York, Harper, 1950.

Van Riper, Charles: *Helping Children to Talk Better.* Better Living Booklets. Chicago, Sci Res Assoc, 1951.

Chapter VI

Ear Training

THE THIRD BASIC REQUIREMENT for a child's language development is ear training. The young baby passes from the babbling stage to a level in language development called lallation. This is a period when the child makes sounds, listens to them, enjoys them, and, therefore, repeats them. It is during this stage that the mother hears her child repeating the sounds *ma ma*. She then asks him to repeat *ma ma*, he listens and she repeats the sounds over and over again until he is able to imitate them. This is ear training. The young child, now able to imitate or "echo" the sounds of others, has entered the "echolalia" stage in his language development. Some children do not develop as fine a sense of sound discrimination as others; some do not develop an adequate memory span for sounds; and some are lacking in both these aspects so important to language growth.

Methods for Initiating Ear Training

1. Remember, it is essential that your child have normal hearing or else amplification to provide him with adequate sound stimulation.

2. Encourage babbling, for it is essential to language acquisition. Play vocally with your child using various sounds to express love, affection, delight, surprise, etc. You may find that it is necessary to use a mirror and to make silent faces first so that the child becomes interested in lip and tongue movements. It is best to start with the *p, b, m,* and *w* sounds with vowels, moving to *t, d, g, k, n* sounds plus vowels when he is able to imitate the more visible bilabial sounds.

3. To aid in the development of auditory perceptual skills, a child should be made aware of environmental sounds. Have your child listen for sounds around the house, such as the vacuum cleaner, the toilet flushing, doorbell ringing, etc. in addition to outdoor sounds (fire siren, airplane, etc.). It might be

44   *Speech and Language Delay*

fun to hide an alarm clock and have him locate the ticking sound. At a higher level, have the child turn his back while you perform an action (bounce a ball, close a door, tear paper, pour water into a jar) and have him identify the action through listening.

4. Reception and understanding of speech sounds are necessary for the development of speech. This requires fine sound discrimination. Training however, must progress from gross to fine listening skills. Take four or five noisemakers (such as a tamborine, child's drum, bell, whistle, and Halloween snapper) and place them on the table in front of the child. Make a noise with each of the noisemakers several times. Next, encourage the child to sound each of the noisemakers. If he is reluctant, help him. Then sound one of the noisemakers and ask him by word or gesture to sound the same noisemaker. Have the child close his eyes or turn his back; again sound a noisemaker and have him open his eyes or turn around. Motion for him to find the noisemaker which you used. The child may require much encouragement, reinforcement of instruction, and actual help at first in carrying out these tasks.

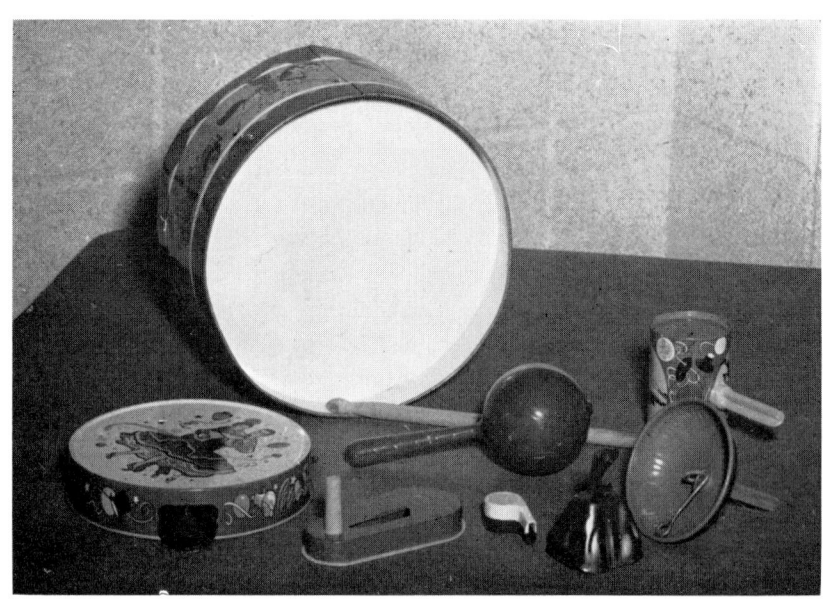

Figure 11. Noisemakers.

Ear Training

5. When the child is able to do the above, he is ready for a slightly more advanced gross-sound drill. You will need two matched sets of four or five similar sounding noisemakers which are only slightly different in pitch or quality. These can be made by partially filling small pill boxes or matchboxes with different ingredients (sand, stones, BB's, glass beads, and pennies). You can also use five shaker-type bells or whistles of similar pitch and quality. Arrange your set and the child's set of noisemakers on the table so that they are in a different order (Fig. 11). Shake, ring, or blow one of your noisemakers while his eyes are closed or he has his back to you. Have the child try to match the sound with a noisemaker from his set. After the child is able to correctly match the noisemakers, make the task more difficult by using a xylophone or piano for the matching game.

6. Listening and rhythm exercises can be fun. Have the child place a block in a box each time you sound a noisemaker (Figs. 12 & 13).

Use noisemakers in playful activities, such as marching, singing, or playing *Simon Says*. Vary the rhythm and see if your child can reproduce the pattern. You can also have your child clap or march to simple tunes.

7. After your child has entered the babbling stage, utilize the sounds which he already *has* in designing nonsense syllables in groups of two or three; use them in a competitive game of imitation. You are not asking for the production of a new sound, but rather, the attention to and retention of an order of sounds already familiar to him. The development of habits of memory will permit him to profit from the everyday speech around him. This is called echolalia and is an important step in language development. Initially, if your child resists auditory stimulation, he may respond to visual stimulation. Therefore, concentrate on giving him visual cues centered around mouth movements. In other words, make faces at him and try to get a similar response.

It is important to note that this drill is not on speech production, but on developing good *listening* habits—beginning speech-sound discrimination and auditory memory for different speech-sound patterns—which allow not only for better understanding

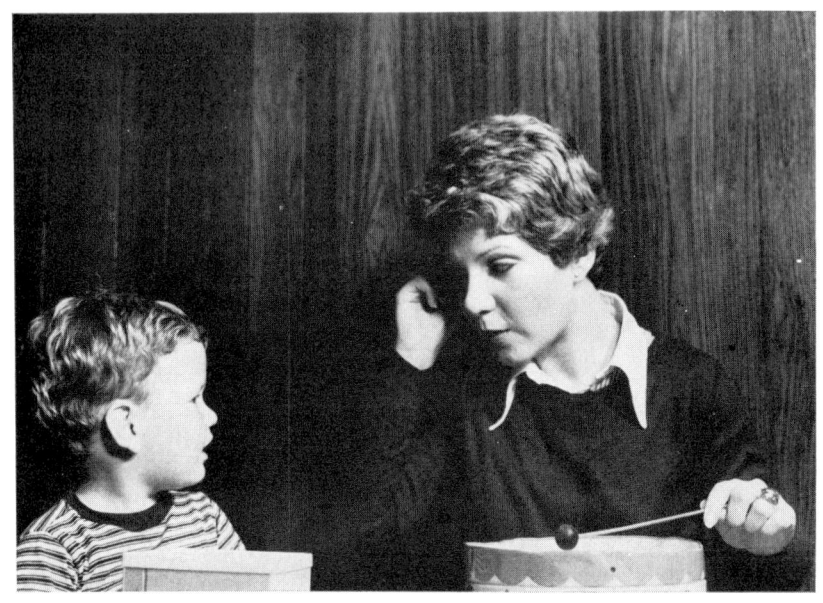

Figure 12. Listening to noisemaker.

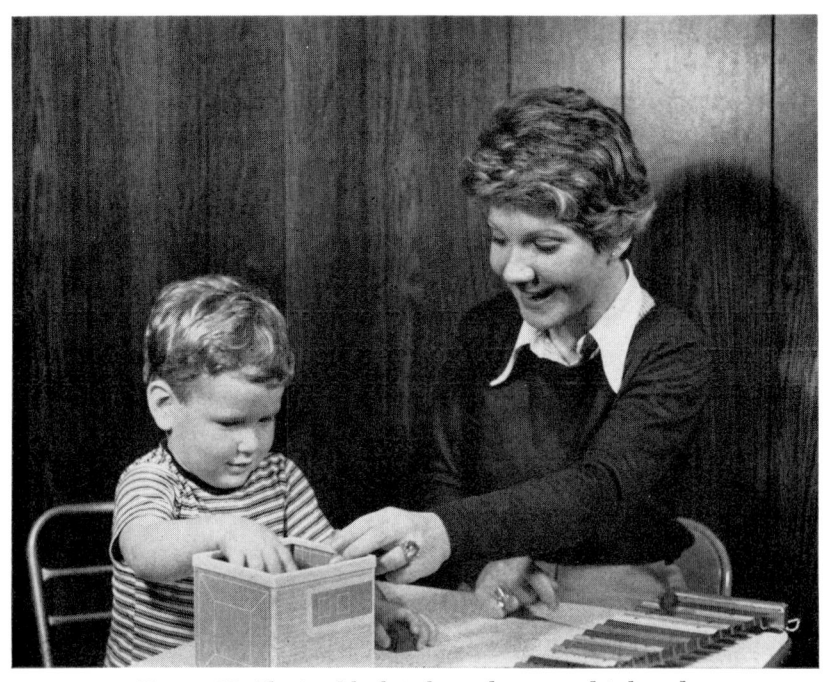

Figure 13. Placing block in box when sound is heard.

Ear Training

but also for better repetition and imitation of speech around the child.

The child delayed in language and speech, even when hearing is normal, typically does not use his auditory-perceptive powers efficiently. Sound, particularly the complex patterns of speech, does not have adequate meaning to the child, and consequently, he attends poorly to the spoken voice. He does not discriminate or "separate out" the individual elements and thus fails to retain patterns of speech-sound combinations. This means that the child finds it difficult to learn speech through repetition of ordinary conversation or even from careful speech stimulation.

For this exercise then, speech sounds should be selected which are within his productive ability. This group usually includes the spoken vowels and the bilabial *(p, b, m, w)*, and sometimes the tongue tip *(t, d, n)* consonants. In this exercise you are not trying to teach the child to say new sounds; you are trying to teach him to attend to the voice carefully, perceive the message accurately, and then hold it in his memory long enough to give it back in exactly the same order in which it was originally given. Thus, a stimulation of $\overline{oo}$, ah, $\overline{e}$, must be repeated $\overline{oo}$, ah, $\overline{e}$, and not $\overline{e}$, ah, $\overline{oo}$, or something else.

Drill begins then with vowels. You may need to start with two vowels, varying their order of presentation. Move to three vowels as quickly as possible. Any three vowels may be chosen and after various orders of presentation are exhausted, one to three other vowels are substituted for a new series.

After success with vowels alone, one of the simple bilabial consonants is used in front of these same vowels making a more difficult series like $\overline{pa}$, $\overline{po}$, $\overline{poo}$, or pah, $\overline{pi}$, pow.

The third order of difficulty of sounds for listening and repeating would be different easy consonants used with the same vowels as in pah, tah, mah or bah, dah, pah. Finally, the most difficult listening and repeating task would be combining various easy consonants with various vowels—for example, t$\overline{ee}$, g$\overline{o}$, bah, or p$\overline{a}$, dah, m$\overline{i}$. When the child is able to repeat accurately these letter combinations in exactly the same order as originally given, he should be ready to better "separate out" spoken sounds. Thus, he can profit from the speech stimulation which goes on about him each day and from which he initially derives little benefit.

In order to keep his attention and interest and motivate him to want to work with you on this game, provide a reward activity which is effective for your particular child. Only thought, imagination, trial and error, and experimentation will establish what the best activities should be. Some possibilities which have proved successful with other children are putting a proffered peg in a pegboard or a marble in a hole in a box each time a listening-repeating task is satisfactorily completed.

Competition games between child and parent are usually exciting and enjoyable. Examples of these might be two ladders drawn on paper which are progressively mounted rung by rung —one for the child when his repetition is correct, one for the parent when he is wrong. Two stick men which are put together one limb or feature at a time may also be used in the same way.

Obtain pairs of small simple toys from the five-and-ten store (such as a car, train, or airplane). Work with one toy at a time.

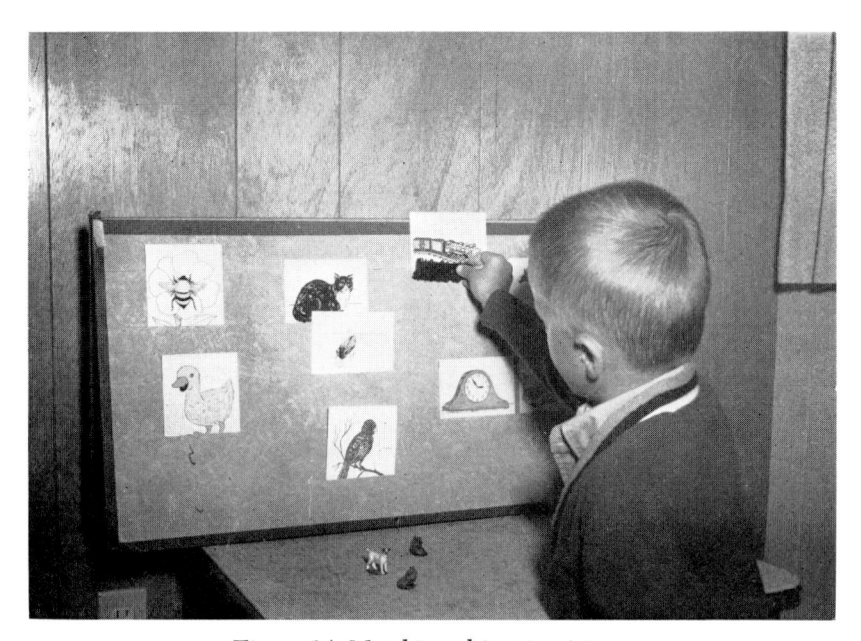

Figure 14. Matching object to picture.

Hold it up near your lips, so that the child can take advantage of the lip movement cues; name the object; hand it to your child; and rename the object as he fingers it.

If it is an object that has a noise associated with it, make the noise as well. For example, the child identifies the cat by touching it or handing it to you when you say "meow." Dog, airplane, car, train, cow, and similar sound-object combinations can be used. You can also play a game where the child matches objects to pictures. You will have to help the child a great deal with the matching in the beginning.

Cut out simple, not overly detailed pictures from magazines or catalogues or purchase word cards from a teacher supply or educational toy store. Be sure there is only one picture on a card. It is wise to get pictures of objects which have sounds as well as a single name associated with them (for example, car—noise of horn or car moving; airplane—noise of motor; cow—moo; cat—meow) (Fig. 15).

    a. Show the cards one at a time to the child.
    b. As you present the card, give the noise associated with the picture and the name.

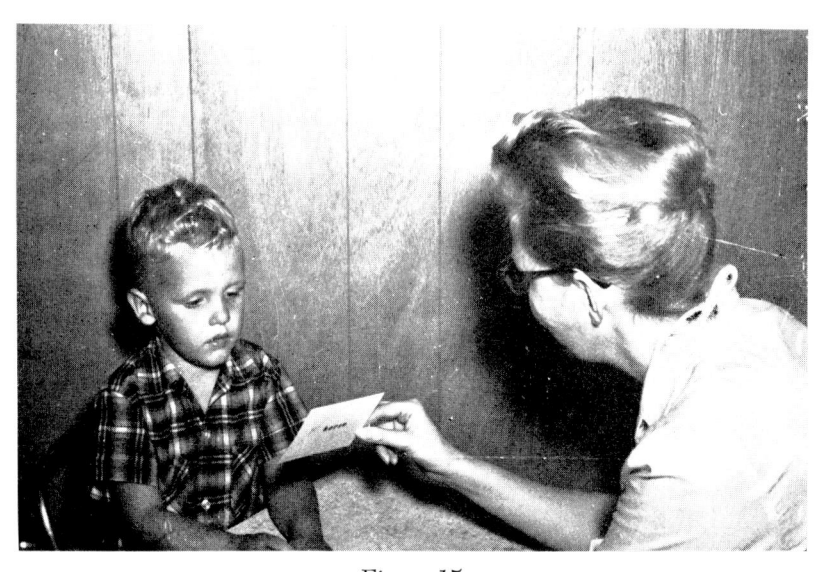

Figure 15

c. Repeat the noise and name many times while talking about the card.
d. Let the child hold the card; then make the noise and take the card from him. Repeat this several times.
e. Make the noise, name the card, and extend your hand for him to give the card to you. Repeat a number of times.
f. Give him several cards which have been used in the previous steps, ask for one by noise and sound, and help him select the correct card and deposit it in your hand. Do this many times.
g. Ask for one of the cards by name and extend your hand for him to give you the correct card.

8. For use with your flannel board, cut simple outline figures from felt such as are shown in Figure 16. At first, use only those figures which have both a name and a sound associated with them. Make the sound such as "moo" for cow, hand the cow to the child, and help him place it on the flannel board. Later name the objects and have him place the figures on the board. Next, place all the felt figures on the flannel board, name one or make its noise, and have the child hand it to you. When the child has acquired a few sounds or words, let him be the teacher and you choose the figures.

9. If the child has difficulty playing *teacher* in number eight, work on imitative word drill. Using either the flannel board figures or picture cards, say one-syllable words and have the child imitate you. Do not be concerned with speech errors, rather, accept close approximations. Reward his imitating attempts by handing him the picture or flannel figure. When he is able to correctly imitate one-syllable words, add pictures with two-syllable names, such as airplane. Remember, consistent drill will result in a *sharper* ear and closer speech approximations.

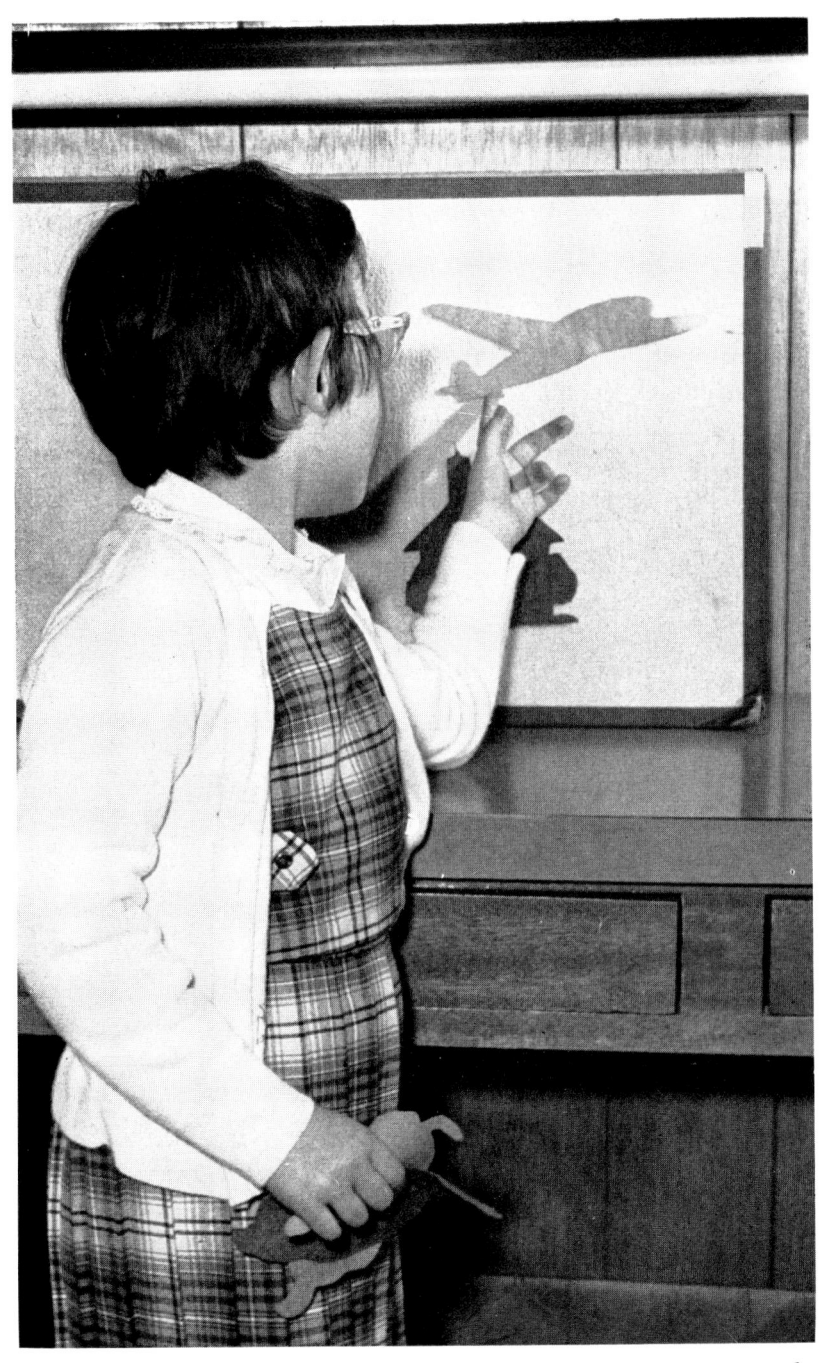

Figure 16. Flannel cutouts for ear training. (Courtesy of Ray Covey, *The Houston Post.*)

Chapter VII

Auditory Perception

THE FOURTH BASIC REQUIREMENT for a language building program is the development of adequate auditory perceptual skills. These include immediate auditory recall, long-term auditory retention, auditory sequential memory, auditory closure, sound blending, and the ability to selectively attend in varying speech/noise environments. Speech authorities have found that many children who are slow in developing speech have poor auditory memory spans—that is, an inability to remember or recall auditory sound patterns. We call this poor verbal imagery. These children have normal hearing and may have good sound discrimination but have, for some reason, little or no ability to retain patterns of auditory stimulation. This poor auditory memory may be the primary factor in the child's failing to develop speech. It also may be partially the result of the speech delay since the child did not have adequate practice in early vocal sound play as described in Chapter I. Thus, a vicious circle may be set up for reinforcement of this poor auditory memory and for further increase in the speech delay.

Children who have a hearing loss will also need training in the development of an adequate auditory memory. These children fail to develop adequate recall for sound patterns and thus for verbal patterns because of their disassociation with a sound environment. Hard-of-hearing children learn to read, to name pictures, and to repeat simple everyday patterned responses, but they have difficulty describing experiences, formulating new ideas, and even participating in simple conversations because they cannot recall verbal patterns unless the response is elicited by a visual clue.

The skills of auditory closure, sound blending, and selective auditory attention are basic for later academic learning. Poor development of these skills may lead to auditory processing and sequencing difficulties such as the following: sounding out words, synthesizing sounds into complete units (c-a-t = cat), following directions, or retaining information long enough to process it.

Ways to Increase Auditory Memory and Retention

1. As you did in ear training, set out five or six noisemakers; ring, tap, or clang two of the instruments one after the other while the child's eyes are closed or his back is turned. Have the child repeat the noises in the same order that they were presented. When he is able to successfully perform this, try three and then four of the noisemakers. He will probably need considerable assistance at first. Be patient and gently assist him to perform the task until he understands what you expect of him and can do it by himself. When the child is able to get four sounds correctly, change the rhythm and time pattern in which the sounds are presented. Start with just one noisemaker and gradually build up to four. Next, try combinations of musical tones on the toy xylophone or piano. First present simple tone combinations and then changes in time and rhythm.

2. Place three or four of the picture cards (discussed in the chapter on ear training) on a table, preferably propped up (Fig. 17). Seat yourself and your child four feet from the table. Name one of the pictures saying "*cow*, bring me the cow," and have your child select the correct picture. Do not repeat the phrase. Vary your voice in loudness and pitch until you find the level to which he responds best. When he is able to correctly select and return with each of the four pictures, add four more pictures to the group. Continue adding to the pictures until the child can correctly select from a group of sixteen.

3. Increase the distance from the table to eight feet and decrease the number of pictures to eight. Repeat the procedure outlined above. Again add pictures by groups of four until you have sixteen pictures.

4. Increase the number of pictures you ask for at a time by two. When the child is able to bring you the sixteen cards correctly in groups of two, request three, then four, and finally five cards.

5. The next step is to remove the visual clues and have the

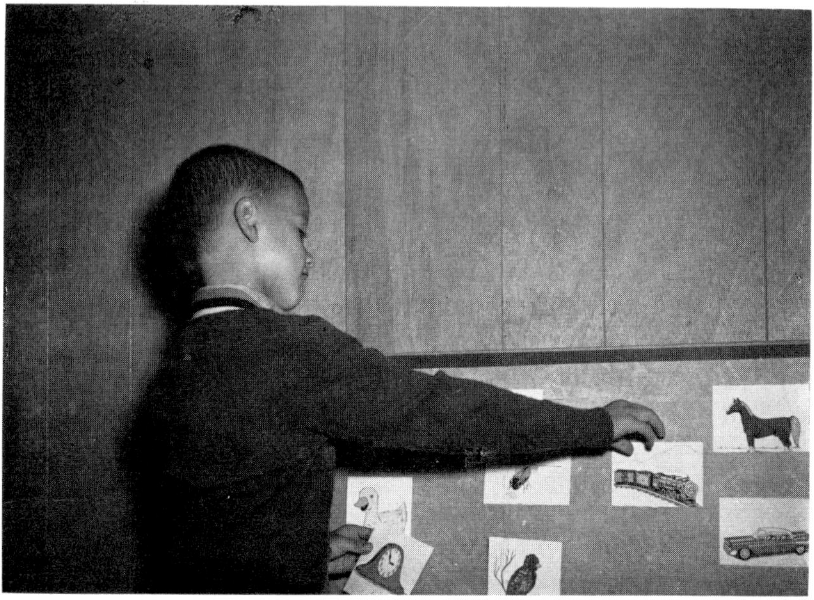

Figure 17. Auditory memory training.

child remember what he has received through auditory means alone. Have him sit about eight feet from the cards and face in the opposite direction. Name three cards and have the child go point to them. When he is able to do this in the correct order, name four and then five cards.

6. Place the cards in the next room and have the child get one, two, three, and finally four cards that you name.

7. Increase the complexity of the request. For example, tell the child to "pick up the *car* and put it under the *chair*." When he is able to carry out correctly the complex requests for a single card, ask for several cards and have him put them in different places. You may also increase the time between your request and his completing the task by having him do something before picking up the cards. (For example, "Walk around the room, then pick up the dog and put it on the window sill.)

8. Place two and then three cards or objects on a table across from where you and the child are seated. He should not be able to see the items. Have him look at them and then come back to

tell you what he saw. If your child has a very limited vocabulary, the items should be within this vocabulary or should have sounds which he can use in place of words.

9. Have your child follow simple instructions which require him to translate the instruction into a motor task. Begin with an easy, single direction such as, "Bring me the *book* from the table." Increase the number and complexity of the tasks according to his ability to achieve. A more difficult set of instructions might include getting an object from another room. For example, "Go to your room, get a black sock, and hide it behind the chair by the fireplace." *Simon Says* and *Follow the Leader* are good memory games. By having the child follow the specific order of the instruction, you not only develop retention and transfer to a motor act but sequencing ability as well.

10. Work to lengthen the amount of time your child can sit and attend by sitting with him while he listens to children's records or watches television. Do not force him to attend beyond the point of his tolerance for the situation; however, each day try to lengthen this *sitting time* slightly. Reading children's books together and playing games can also be used. Remember, unless highly motivated, a child's attention span is his age plus five. Therefore, if your child is three years old, his attention should approximate eight minutes.

11. Once some success has been achieved in auditory-memory development, encourage, reward, reinforce, and participate actively and enthusiastically in all attempts by the child to commit any verbal messages to memory. Also participate in recitation of these memorized items whether they be poems, nursery rhymes, jingles, children's tunes or hit songs, commercials, and sayings or expressions. Many television commercials are particularly appealing to young children and are available; they are also sufficiently repetitive and reinforced to be a very effective source of stimulation for this activity. Do not be inhibited or self-conscious in this memory work. Take an active role, dramatize the material, and have fun with your child whether you are listening to him recite, praising his efforts, or saying the material for or with him.

Advanced Listening Activities

1. Place two objects or pictures on the table. Name one item omitting a part of the word and have the child point to that item. For example, "ba..y" (child points to *baby*), "pu..y" (puppy), "coo..ie" (cookie). Increase the number of pictures from which the child must choose.

2. Place two common pictures cards on the table. Say the individual sounds of the word and have the child point to the picture; for example "c-a-t" (child points to *cat*). Increase the number of pictures from which the child chooses to four, then six, then eight as he is able to handle the task. Never advance to the larger set until the child is capable of meeting with some success.

3. Both of the above activities can be made more difficult by removing the visual cues and having the child say the word. Select words from his speaking vocabulary. These activities are more difficult and you will need to allow your child to practice until he understands what is expected of him.

4. Noise makes even the simplest listening task harder. Gradually condition your child to pay attention in the presence of noise.

    a. Have the child complete easy fun tasks (coloring, block building, puzzle completion, finger painting) with noise in the background. Use a radio, stereo, television, or family chatter as your source of noise. Help your child center his attention on the task while he *tunes out* the competing messages or sounds. This may be very difficult for both you and your child and will require much patience on your part.

    b. Play the radio very softly while talking to your child. Can he pay attention to what you are saying? Can he follow directions? Work to increase the length of attention with a minimal amount of noise present.

    c. Perform already mastered auditory activities in the presence of the television, radio, stereo, or people talking. Keep these activities simple as you increase the amount of background noise. Previously difficult activities with noise may be frustrating for the child. In fact, many school-age children have not developed the ability to filter out classroom noises while attending to the teacher. This can lead to later learning deficits.

Chapter VIII

Visual Perception

VISUAL PERCEPTION is the fifth and last basic requirement of a language building program. This category includes visual memory, visual closure, and visual discrimination. Visual memory is the ability to remember what we see. This ability includes remembering the shape of what we see, its relationship to other things in the environment, its direction or position in space, and the order in which we see it. This latter ability is called visual sequencing and is particularly important to spelling, reading, and arithmetic ability when a child is older. It is vital to the child with a hearing loss for the development of lipreading skills.

Just as form perception or the ability to separate foreground from background is a part of language, so is the ability to remember what we see and the order in which we see it. Eisenson at Stanford University made a detailed study of children with severe language delay and found the subjects were severely depressed in sequencing ability, both auditory and visual. Battin and Kraft studied school-age children with learning and behavior problems and found a high percentage of these children depressed in visual-sequencing ability. We have learned that sequencing ability can be taught; when a child is depressed in this area, training brings improvement.

Visual closure is the ability to perceive and integrate a complete object or form when only parts are presented. This skill is needed to be able to piece together a puzzle, connect dotted pictures or simply to integrate our environment, to know the wall extends behind the couch or the floor under the table. Visual discrimination is the ability to perceive likenesses and differences in visually presented materials. A lack of awareness in these areas could result in reading misperceptions: (cat–cot; sing–ring; was–saw), punctuation errors, and spelling difficulties.

Until recently, children with learning difficulties were not identified until they reached the fourth or fifth grade. By that time, these children had met repeated failure and had become defeated. In an attempt to catch these children at a younger age, before they had developed a poor self-image and a sense of failure, and before poor learning habits had been established, a detailed study was made of development and behavior patterns. A high percentage of these children had a history of severe language or speech delay or both. They were described by parents and teachers in the following terms: having a short attention span, being hyperactive, not having the ability to follow directions, being easily distracted, being unable to complete the task at hand, and being easily frustrated. These descriptions also fit many of our younger children with speech and language delay. Therefore, in an attempt to circumvent visual perceptual problems in later years, we have included visual perceptual training in our language program.

Supplies Needed for Visual Training

1. Several small toys, e.g. car, dog, truck, cat, doll, airplane
2. Small cardboard box which will completely and easily cover each of the above-named toys
3. Flannel board and felt figures
4. Colored blocks
5. Pegboard and pegs
6. Colored pipe cleaners
7. Crayons, pencils, and paper
8. Blackboard and chalk
9. Plastic clay
10. Infant's large wooden beads for stringing, and two large shoelaces
11. Puzzles
12. Simple pictures
13. Pictures containing hidden objects
14. Connect the dot pictures
15. Stencils

Ways to Increase Visual Memory, Visual Closure, and Visual Discrimination

1. PLAYING WITH BLOCKS. Building blocks can be used to develop memory, sequencing, and spatial relations. Have your child copy simple designs or structures that you build. For example, a three-block tower, three-block bridge, four-block train or similar simple designs. Be sure to name what you build and to assign some action to it (such as knocking down the tower, pushing something under the bridge, pushing the train and making the whistle noise).

2. COPYING A BEAD CHAIN. First, allow your child to copy a simple pattern that you have made with the large primary beads.

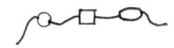

When he can copy the design easily, see if he can produce a bead pattern from memory. Start with two beads and build to four or five.

3. PUZZLES. Puzzles are very helpful in strengthening visual sequencing and closure skills, in addition to developing fine motor coordination (Fig. 18). If a puzzle appears too difficult, remove only a part of the pieces. The remaining pieces will assist the child in perceiving the whole.

4. COPYING SIMPLE DESIGNS ON THE PEGBOARD. Place the pegs in a row working from left to right. Use only a few at first and limit the number of colors to two or three. Have your child copy the color design immediately under your row of pegs. Be sure he works from left to right. As mentioned previously, increase the difficulty by having the child reproduce a peg pattern from memory.

5. USE OF OBJECTS OR PICTURES. Place three small toys or pictures in front of your child, have him look at them for several seconds, then have him close his eyes. Cover one of the items with the small box; have him look at the remaining items and

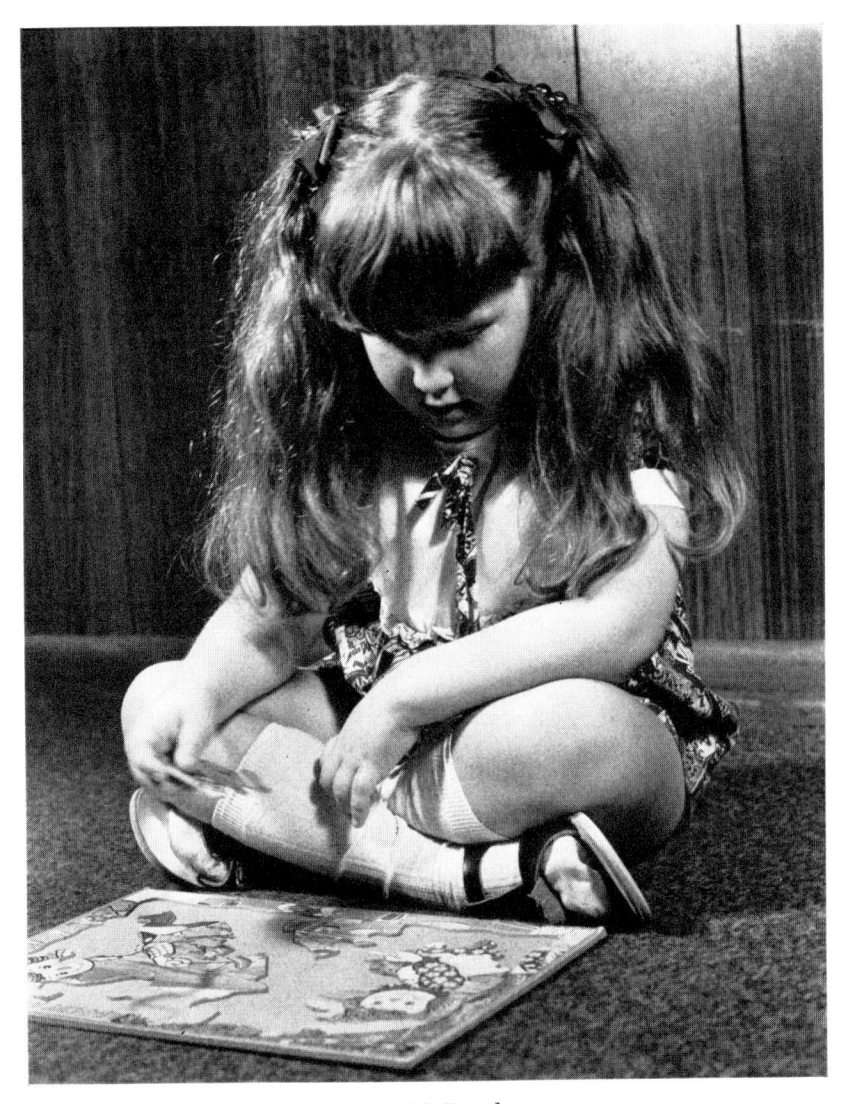

Figure 18. Puzzles.

tell you (either through words, sounds, or gestures) what is missing. Gradually increase the number of items you use to five or six, and cover two of them. When the child is able to do this easily, place three toys or pictures before him. Next have him cover his eyes while you mix up the toys. Then have him open his eyes and replace the items in the proper order. Vary the task by asking the child if he can recall all of the items hidden under the box.

6. Use of the Flannel Board. Repeat the above procedure, but use felt objects on the flannel board in place of toys (Fig. 19). Remember this is a visual task so do not name the objects when you place them on the flannel board. This will be similar to what you did in auditory memory but the auditory clues will have been removed.

7. Use your felt circle, triangle, cross and square on the flannel board and have your child copy the order in which you arrange them with his own felt figures. However, have him place his figures on the table. This then becomes a more difficult task since he must translate what he sees on the upright flannel board to a flat surface. This is important preparation for school.

8. Matching and Sorting. Using a duplicate set of pictures, toys, or flannel figures, have the child match a sequence of items placed before him. Matching objects to their respective pictures becomes a more complex task. Have the child sort blocks according to color and buttons according to size, i.e. all green blocks to-

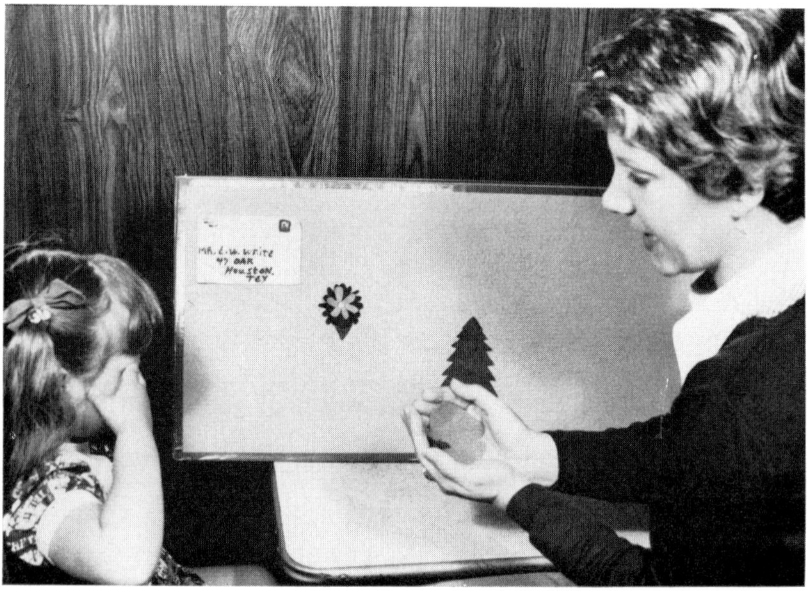

Figure 19. Visual memory training.

Visual Perception 63

gether, etc. At a higher level, have the child match printed letters, numbers, or shapes.

9. Use toothpicks or make thin felt bars ½ inch by 3 inches. Place them on the table in front of your child in a simple design.

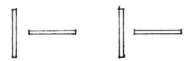

|— |—

Have him copy the design with pipe cleaners. Gradually increase the complexity of the design but keep the bars separated by an inch.

/\ |_ ⌐|

Next place the flannel bars on the flannel board and have him copy them with pipe cleaners. When the designs are copied with ease, begin to place the bars closer together until eventually each design is made of complete units.

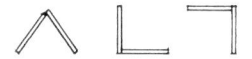

△ L ⌐

10. If your child has difficulty copying the designs with the pipe cleaners, try using clay. Roll the clay into long, thin strips and twist and turn it into different patterns. You have added touch to the task and made it easier.

11. Copying written or printed material is more difficult. Repeat your felt designs by drawing them on the blackboard. Again separate them about an inch between the joints. First, have your child copy them with clay, pipe sticks, or both; then have him try it on a slate or with large crayons, and finally with pencil and paper. Gradually bring the parts of the design units together as you did with the flannel board.

12. Place a piece of tracing paper over a page in a coloring book. Have the child trace the picture and then color it.

13. Use simple dot to dot designs. See if he can guess the picture before the dots are connected.

14. Drawing is related to visual sequencing. As your child improves in visual sequencing and retention ability, his drawings will begin to show improvement. Help him by starting a drawing and letting him complete it or use dots as a guide for him to follow.

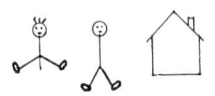

15. Utilize magazines and newspaper items in which the child is to find hidden pictures. *Highlights* and other children's magazines are excellent sources.

16. Purchase or make stencils for the child to trace. Overlap two stencils and see if he can discriminate the two pictures. Increase the number of figures as his ability improves. Have your child outline each item in a different color.

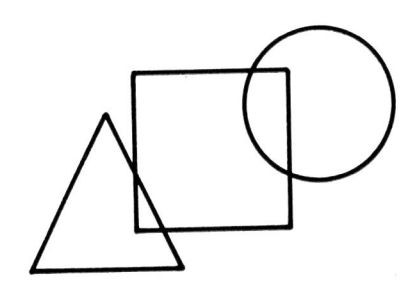

17. Hide familiar objects such as shoes, balls, mittens, etc. about the room. Allow only a small portion of the object to be in view. See how quickly he can find all of the objects.

18. USE YOUR IMAGINATION. Just remember, keep tasks simple and relate them to your other language activities.

Chapter IX

The Hard-of-Hearing Child

ALTHOUGH THE HARD-OF-HEARING child will need the five basic requirements for the development of speech and language mentioned in the previous chapters, he will also require some special considerations. First, it will be necessary to establish the presence of a hearing loss through careful, repeated observations of failure to respond to sound.

It will be necessary to have the child examined by a physician, preferably an otolaryngologist, and to have his hearing tested by an audiologist. This testing will establish whether a hearing loss is present and if so, the extent and the nature of the loss. This information, together with the history and physical examination, will permit the physician to diagnose the problem and to prescribe medical treatment, a hearing aid, or both. If a hearing aid is indicated, the audiologist will determine which hearing aid and which adjustments of the aid are most suitable for the child. He will provide guidance in the care of the aid, adjustment to its wear, and counsel regarding special schools and home training programs for language and speech development, auditory training, and speechreading.

The hearing testing of the young child, particularly the preschool child, is a very specialized art requiring highly skilled audiologists with graduate training and experience in pediatric audiology, sophisticated instrumentation and a good deal of time and patience. With the above set of conditions, children can be successfully tested down to six months of age. This testing is often accomplished by some form of behavioral orientation conditioning in which the infant or young preschooler is trained to turn to high volume pure tone sound from a loudspeaker by being rewarded with a bright light and puppet in a usually darkened window (Figs. 20 & 21). Sounds are then lowered in intensity gradually until the threshold of hearing is established. After this stage, earphone testing progresses in the

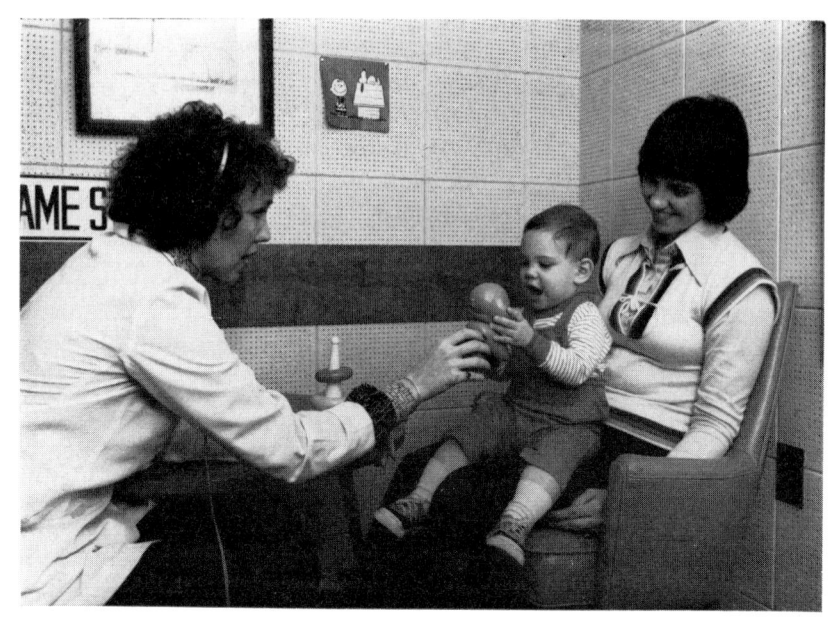

Figure 20. Twelve-month-old, hard-of-hearing child being tested with the PIWI technique with loudspeaker stimulation. Attention fixed on playing with toys.

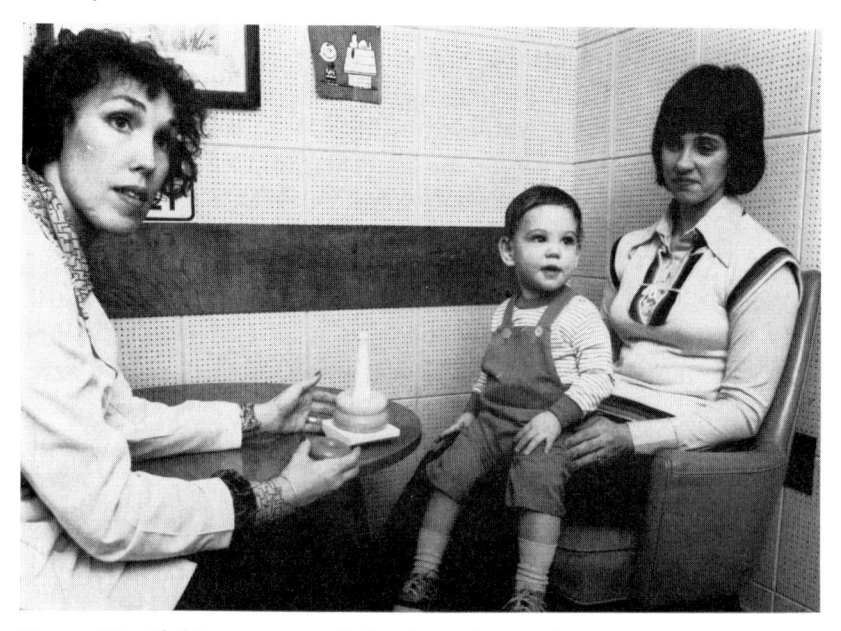

Figure 21. Child turning to lighted window and puppet in response to sound from loudspeaker.

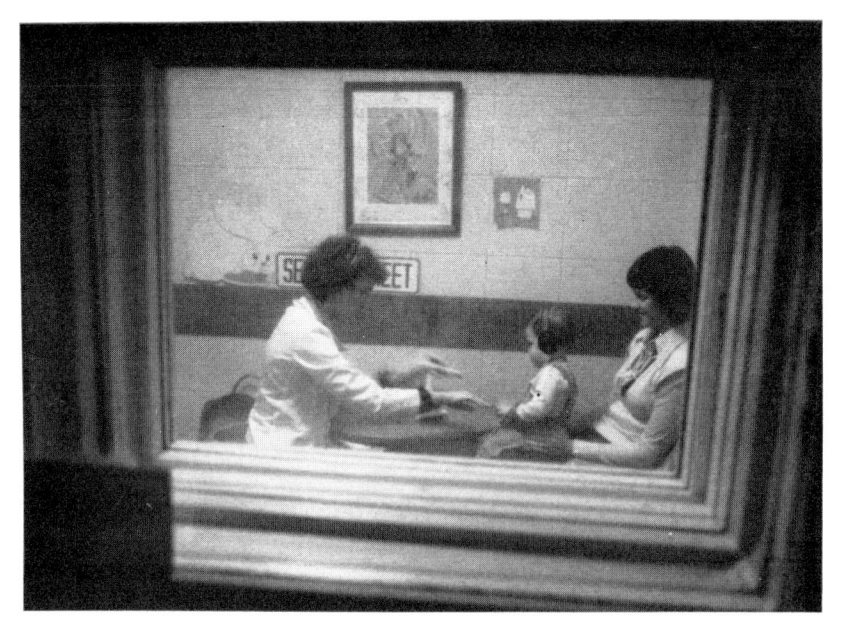

Figure 22. Twelve-month-old child being tested with PIWI technique using earphones. Attention focused on toys on table.

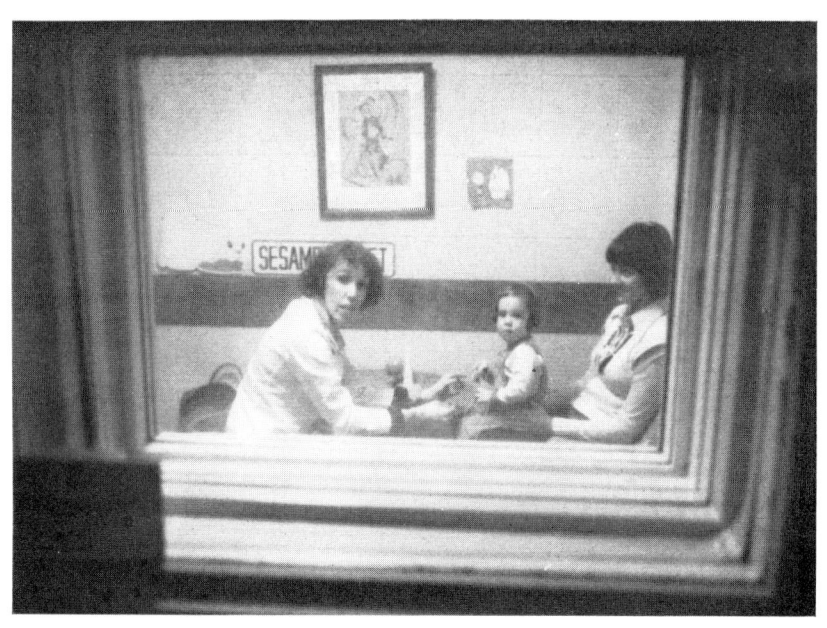

Figure 23. Child responding by turning to puppet in window illuminated (PIWI), after hearing a pure tone through the earphones.

68 *Speech and Language Delay*

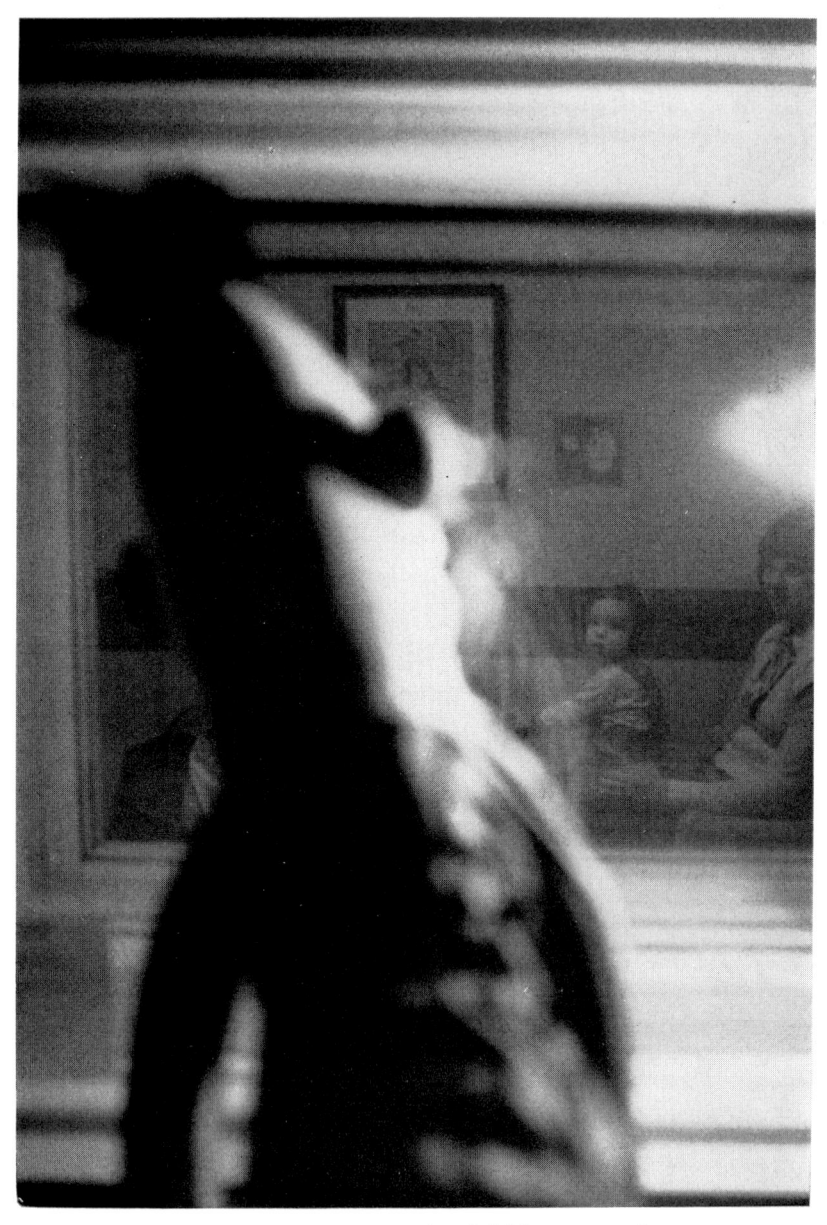

Figure 24. Puppet seen by child being tested.

same manner to establish hearing thresholds for each ear (Figs. 22, 23, 24). Following this, mastoid bone conduction is measured in order to establish the type of loss present and the condition of the hearing nerve. If a hearing aid is worn, thresholds may now be obtained with the hearing aid. If a comparison of instruments evaluation is to be done, this testing is usually put off to a second visit in order not to overtire the child.

This type of conditioning testing does not require speech or verbal understanding by the child. Pure tone thresholds and voice awareness can all be measured by gesture, expression, and reward. If the child has speech understanding, even without speech use, he can more easily be tested for pure tones and his speech reception threshold measured by pointing to pictures of two-syllable spondee type words. Studies correlating the hearing test findings before and after ear surgery with the history and physical ear findings before, at the time of surgery, and after, have established high validity of real threshold levels of these young children. Test-retest measurements on permanent sensori-neural type losses have established good reliability of these measurements as well.

Some of the criteria used to evaluate the success and reliability of a given test on young children are these:
1. Appropriateness and timing of the responses in relation to the stimulation.
2. Consistency of response of various trials at threshold.
3. Correlation between thresholds by loudspeaker and those of the better ear by earphone.
4. Agreement between the pure tone averages and the speech reception or speech awareness thresholds.

When lack of proper equipment, technique, or cooperation on the part of the very young child precludes getting a valid, reliable measure of the child's hearing by behavioral response, the audiologist may do a prediction of the approximate hearing sensitivity levels by objective responses obtained to acoustic reflex testing called Sensitivity Prediction from Acoustic Reflex (SPAR) or to Electric Response Audiometry (either Brain Stem Evoked Response (BSER) or Electro-Cochleography (ECOG).

If testing discloses a hearing loss which is determined to be irreversible by medical or surgical means, a hearing aid evaluation or selection should be done, again preferably by a clinical audiologist. The audiologist will compare suitable aids to determine the best performing instrument for the particular child involved. If this comparison is unreliable because of the age of the child, a suitable aid, with all settings and fitting specifications, will be prescribed for trial. With the young child, a hearing aid trial period should always be sought, before actual purchase takes place, because a given child may sometimes reject an aid completely on first approach, but be quite willing to accept it in a later trial, three to six months later. Recent advances in hearing aid technology now make it possible for many children with moderately severe to severe hearing losses to be reached by high gain over-the-ear type instruments. Often these will have external receivers of a CROS type fitting which puts the receiver on the opposite side of the head from the microphone, permitting control of feedback squeal. The most severe to profound losses will still best be fitted with one of the very powerful body type instruments (Fig. 25).

If binaural fitting is to be used, that is a hearing aid for each ear, it should be with two completely separate instruments rather than one unit with a "Y" cord split to each ear. The "Y" cord arrangement limits the individual ear fitting possibilities and unless special resistance receivers are used, power will be significantly reduced over single-ear fitting.

Lipreading and Auditory Discrimination Suggestions

The hard-of-hearing child must learn to use all his senses so that he can supplement the stimuli he receives through the impaired-hearing mechanism. In addition, the child must learn to receive maximum benefit from the hearing that he has. The following suggestions should be used in addition to the material in the previous chapters.

1. Do not shout if the child is wearing his hearing aid. You are overloading the aid and causing distortion. In addition, the increased loudness may actually be painful.

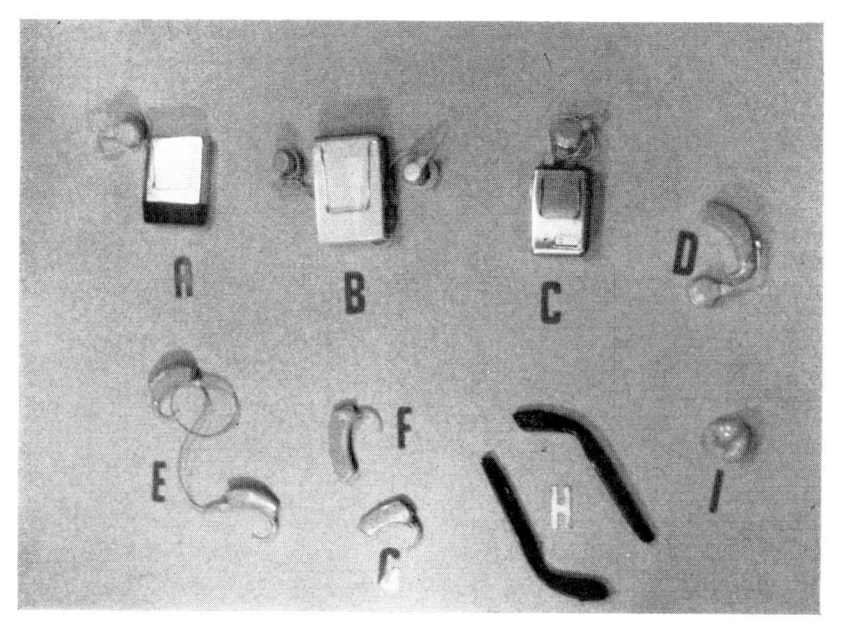

Figure 25. Types of hearing aids. A. Power body aid—for most severe losses. B. Binaural power body aids in one case—for severe losses. C. Regular body aid—for moderate to moderately severe losses. D. Power over ear with external receiver—for severe losses. E. Power CROS over ear—for severe losses. F. Power over ear with internal receiver—for moderately severe losses. G. Regular over ear with internal receiver—for moderate losses. H. Power CROS glasses—for severe losses. I. All-in-ear suitable only for mild to moderate losses primarily.

2. Look directly at the child when you are talking to him.

3. When you talk, do not cover up your mouth with a book, a newspaper, or with your hands.

4. Do not speak with a cigar, a cigarette, or a pipe in your mouth.

5. Hold your head still and steady when speaking.

6. Adjust your position so that the light—whether from lamp or window—is on your face, not on the child's face.

7. Speak slowly.

8. Speak distinctly with an active mouth. Do not slur or mumble.

9. If the child fails to get your meaning, rephrase or reword, as well as repeat what you have said.

10. Be patient.

11. Remember that lipreading and listening go together, and one never interferes with the other.

12. Encourage the child to look at the speaker's mouth at all times so that he sees the lip position of the words as he hears them.

13. Help the child to investigate or find the sources of all new sounds. Tell him the name of the object or animal which is making the sounds as he hears and sees it.

14. After the child has learned to identify sounds, play "eyes covered" games in which he must tell you or show you the sound heard.

15. Talk, talk, talk to the child all day long about familiar objects and everyday actions at the same time that he sees them. Do not worry if he does not seem to be paying attention; if he does not understand or does not say the words, just keep talking. If you talk enough to give him something to say—and to give him the opportunity to improve his listening and looking—he too will start talking.

16. As you teach young children the names of things, bring the picture or object up close to your mouth whenever possible so that he can see lips form the word as he sees the object.

17. Have the child pick up objects as you say the names—first with watching your lips and listening, and then with listening alone.

18. Have the child listen to difficult words and word pairs that sound alike, identifying what he has heard (for example, bat-cat, shoe-two, tie-pie, cap-cup, bed-bread).

Care of the Hearing Aid Instrument

1. Do not leave it where it can be overheated.

2. Do not allow it to become wet or exposed to excessive moisture. If the aid does become wet:
    a. Sling out water by vigorous shaking.
    b. Blot up with blotter or absorbent paper.

The Hard-of-Hearing Child

    c. Wrap it in absorbent tissue.

    d. Bring it in to the hearing aid dealer as soon as possible.

3. Do not drop (handle like a delicate electronic instrument).

4. Do not bend, twist, or snag the cord, if it has one.

5. Do not wear the hearing aid when engaged in active play, or sports, where it could be struck or dislodged and damaged.

6. Do not use hair spray on the child's hair while the hearing aid is being worn.

7. Turn off the aid and open the battery compartment at night or when the aid is not in use.

8. Keep a spare cord on hand (if aid uses a cord), and replace when the sound cuts off and on.

9. Keep spare batteries on hand, and replace them when the aid does not function, or when the power is weak.

10. Parents should listen to the hearing aid each morning to note any humming, buzzing, static, or any other unusual sounds.

11. Wipe off the earpiece periodically to clean it and remove wax from the sound opening with a toothpick. It is better not to remove the earpiece from the tubing. Let your dealer do that.

12. Several times a week do these things to reduce the build-up of corrosion or when the aid does not work properly:

    a. Rub the battery ends with a rubber pencil eraser, rough cloth or sole of the shoe.

    b. Do the same with the battery compartment contacts.

    c. Rotate the tone control (if present) back and forth rapidly.

    d. Rotate the volume control back and forth rapidly.

    e. While holding the heavy tip, pull the cord (if it has one) in and out of the amplifier.

    f. Do the same with the other end of the cord which fits on the receiver button.

13. When putting in the battery or batteries, line up the + (positive) end of the battery with the + (positive) end of the battery compartment.

14. Each time the hearing aid is put on, be sure that the earpiece is firmly seated in the ear and that the volume of the hear-

ing aid is not on full gain in order to prevent feedback squealing.

15. When the aid is not being worn in the ear, and the volume is turned up, it is normal for it to squeal.
- a. If squealing occurs frequently while the hearing aid is being worn, check the following:
    - (1) See that the earpiece is firmly seated in the ear.
    - (2) See that the volume has not been turned up to maximum.
    - (3) See that the wearer is not seated in a corner or up close to a hard, reflecting surface.
    - (4) See that the wearer's hand is not being cupped close to the hearing aid or to the ear, when adjusting the aid.
- b. If the above have been checked and feedback squealing continues when the aid is worn, make the following tests:
    - (1) Turn the hearing aid up to the normal comfortable setting and place the thumb tightly over the earpiece opening. If squealing is heard, there is a sound leak somewhere. Have your dealer check the aid.
    - (2) If no squealing occurs on the above test, by process of elimination, the trouble must be that the earpiece is too small or poorly fitted. See your dealer about a new, tighter fitting earpiece.

16. High humidity often causes moisture to be a problem in hearing aid wear. These suggestions should be helpful in this regard.
- a. Do not blow moisture out of your aid, receiver, tubing or earpiece. That may only cause the deposit of additional moisture. Use a rubber bulb syringe to blow it out.
- b. Use a silica gel air dryer in a plastic bag or box to put the aid in at night for drying by absorption of moisture. Get this material from your hearing aid dealer.

Placing the Hearing Aid in the Ear

1. Take hold of the outer ear in back and pull it outwards and downwards, with one hand. With the other hand, guide the

top of the earpiece into the notch or groove above the canal. Push the earpiece canal tip part into the ear canal and the large rounded part of the earpiece down into the hollows of the ear until it slips into place and becomes "part of the ear" and feels comfortable and tight.

2. An alternative method is to insert the earpiece canal tip into the ear canal, pointing the upper tip of the earpiece toward the patient's eye. Then rotate the earpiece backward until the small uppermost tip of the earpiece slips into the front notch above and forward of the ear canal, the whole earpiece settles into the hollow of the ear and feels comfortable.

Adjustments to the Wearing of the Hearing Aid

1. Have the child wear the aid for several days indoors in quiet surroundings. Have him talk to only one or two persons at a time. Keep the aid on him for short periods of thirty minutes to one hour. Keep the volume slightly lowered at first.

2. For several days, introduce a controlled noise and sound background by turning on the radio, record player, or television while talking to the child. Lengthen the periods of wearing the aid and increase the volume.

3. Next, have the child wear the aid from several days to a week in all situations indoors. Have him wear it all day. Increase the volume to about three-fourths gain or to a comfortable level for his hearing of your voice. This level should be below the feedback squeal point.

4. Finally, have the child wear the aid in all difficult situations, indoors and outdoors.

REFERENCES

Biebe, H. H.: *A Guide to Help the Severely Hard of Hearing Child*. New York, S. Karger, 1953.

Consumer's Guide: *Facts about Hearing and Hearing Aids*. Washington, National Bureau of Standards. U. S. Department of Commerce.

Editor: *Correspondence Course for Parents of Preschool Deaf and Hard-of-Hearing Children*. Los Angeles, John Tracy Clinic, 806 Adams Blvd., Los Angeles, California.

Downs, Marion P.: The Establishment of Hearing Aid Use; A Program for Parents, *Maico Audiological Library Series*, Vol. IV, 1967.

Haug, Olaf, Baccaro, Paul and Guilford, Frederick R.: A Pure-Tone Audiogram on the Infant, the PIWI Technique. *Archives of Otolaryngology,* 86:435-440, 1967.

Hodgson, W. R.: Testing Infants and Young Children. In Katz, J. (Ed.): *Handbook of Clinical Audiology.* Baltimore, Williams and Wilkins, 1972.

Lassman, Grace: *Language for the Preschool Deaf Child.* New York, Grune, 1950.

Miller, M. H. and Polisar, I. A.: *Audiological Evaluation of the Pediatric Patient.* Springfield, Thomas, 2nd Printing, 1971.

Moffat, S.: *Helping the Child Who Cannot Hear.* New York. The Public Affairs Committee, Public Affairs Pamphlet No. 479, 1972.

Myklebust, Helmer E. L.: *Your Deaf Child.* Springfield, Thomas, 1960.

Northern, Jerry L. and Downs, Marion P.: *Hearing in Children.* Baltimore, Williams and Wilkins, 1974.

Pollack, D.: *Educational Audiology for the Limited Hearing Infant.* Springfield. Thomas, 1970.

Ronnei, E.: *Learning to Look and Listen.* New York, Bureau of Publications, Teachers College, Columbia University, 1951.

Silverman, S. R. and Lane, H. S.: Deaf Children. In Davis, H. and Silverman, S. R. (Eds.): *Hearing and Deafness,* 3rd ed. New York, H, R & W, 1970.

Tracy, Richmond et al.: *If You Have a Deaf Child.* Urbana, U of Ill Pr, 1959.

Utley, Jean: *What's Its Name.* Urbana, U of Ill Pr, 1950. (Auditory Training Album Optional.)

Chapter X

Is My Child Ready for First Grade?

CULTURALLY, it has become tradition in this country, as well as in many European countries, for a youngster to enter first grade at or during his sixth year. Many parents are upset when their child's sixth birthday falls a few days short of allowing him to enter first grade. They bemoan the fact that their child will be "almost seven" before he enters the primary grades. We are in error when we use chronological age as the gauge for school readiness.

Children mature in different skills at different rates, and it is maturation of basic skills which should be the determining factor for entrance into a formal educational program. At the time of this writing, in Texas, a father is suing the state because his exceptionally bright, five-year-old girl is not permitted to attend second grade (where she is placed according to academic achievement) for a full school day. The public school refuses to allow the youngster to attend for more than a half day because the state only reimburses the school district for a half day for five-year-old youngsters. The ramifications of this case will have far-reaching consequences should the father win his case, for as long as chronological age is used as a criteria for school services rendered, other parents will demand equal time and five-year-old children of normal learning skills will be pushed into attending a formalized program for a full day.

At the other extreme, some specialists believe academic training should be postponed until after a child's seventh birthday. There is some evidence that a child can be withheld from school until his ninth birthday and he will catch up to his peers in approximately nine weeks of school.

What does all this mean to the parents? How can they know what is best for their child? Research conducted by Piaget (Institute des Sciences d'Education, Universite de Geneve, Switzerland) suggests that children internally integrate certain facts from their environment around age seven when facts are critical to academic learning. At age seven, a child is able to recognize or tell whether objects have the same quantities, i.e. a piece of clay formed into a ball and then formed into a long, skinny snake has maintained the same amount of clay, that is, nothing was added or taken away. However, he will be ten or older before he realizes that the ball and the snake displace the same amount of water or that they weigh the same. Can these concepts or experiences be taught? No, for they do not make sense to the average seven- or eight-year-old, they are too abstract.

If, then, certain concepts or experiences cannot be taught or internalized, what does a child acquire in the first grade that he could not have acquired as well at home? Perhaps the answer is socialization, increase in attention span, and the beginnings of a specific form of self-discipline. That is, the egocentric youngster learns to conform to external pressures of teacher and peers.

The following are speech and language developmental skills that your child should have acquired before first grade readiness is considered to have been reached:

1. He should be able to talk freely and clearly with articulation development (speech understandability) better than 90 percent.
2. He should be able to understand and follow simple oral directions.
3. The numerical size of his vocabulary should be greater than 1500 words.
4. His sentence length should be at least four words.
5. He should know his colors and four or five prepositions.
6. He should know most common opposites.
7. He should use past and future verb tenses, comparatives, adjectives, and adverbs.
8. In communication he should be able to relate experiences as well as seek information.
9. He should ask permission, give excuses, and know to say please and thank you.
10. He should be able to give his full name and address.
11. Attention should have increased to where the child can

be reached by auditory and visual stimulation and can complete activities begun.
12. He should be able to recognize likenesses and differences in size, color, shape, texture, and in letters, sounds, and word forms.
13. He should use left to right eye movement in looking at sequential pictures.
14. He should use left to right sequence in making a series of pictures.
15. He should be able to relate a personal experience in the order in which it occurred.
16. He should show an interest in books, labels, and signs.
17. He should enjoy listening to stories and poems.
18. He should indicate a desire to read.
19. He should be able to recite the alphabet.
20. He should be able to recite a four-line poem or nursery rhyme, count to ten, count four objects, and repeat four digits.
21. He should have developed some sense of spatial orientation.

If he is not able to do most of these things, do not push him into first grade just because his chronological age qualifies him. Rather, intensify your home training efforts at language stimulation, motivation, and ear training; give him professional language development training and enroll or re-enroll him in nursery school or kindergarten.

REFERENCES

Flavell, John H.: *The Developmental Psychology of Jean Piaget.* New York, Van Nostrand Reinhold Co., 1963.

Kraft, I. and Battin, R. Ray: The Under Achiever. *Journal of the American Medical Women's Association,* July, pp. 343-348, 1973.

Meier, John H.: Learning Disabilities Found in the Schools. In Satz, Paul and Ross, John L. (Eds.): *The Disabled Learner.* Groningen, Rotterdam U Pr, 1972.

Webber, Robert E.: Early Childhood Development. In Webber, Robert E. (Ed.): *Handbook on Learning Disabilities.* Englewood Cliffs, P-H, Inc., 1974.

Chapter XI

The Parent as a Teacher

IN THE PRECEDING PAGES, we have set out a course of action for parents to follow so that they can assist the child in the development of speech and language. In doing this, we have assumed that they can don the cloak of a teacher at times and still maintain the role of a parent. Although parents are continually teaching their children, their approach to the child is different from that of a teacher. The emotional response of parents to their child's success or failure, their pleasure in the child's achievement, their feelings of love, pride, and disappointment are different from those of a teacher. The teacher is attempting to view the child in an objective manner so that she can measure his needs and accomplishments. In this way, the teacher structures her lessons to meet the needs of the child. Parents, on the other hand, have difficulty in assuming this objective attitude; their own emotions are interlaced with their evaluation of the child. Such feelings as fear, embarrassment, rejection, and apprehension color the reaction of the parent to the child's abilities and accomplishments.

It is important that parents of children with a handicap accept the problem. They should be convinced and try to convince their child that he can succeed *not in spite of* his handicaps but *because of* them. He does this by developing habits of unusual efforts and by taking more advantage of his other capabilities. Parents should remember:

> To learn is a joy;
> To teach is a joy—
> And a privilege.

Parents of a handicapped child sometimes give this child too much attention and thus sacrifice or neglect other members of the family. All children must grow up being a part of the family circle and must learn to accept and share equally in the responsibilities, joys, accomplishments, failures, and disappointments that go with being a member of a family. It is important to remember that the child with a speech and language delay or with any handicap *needs as much opportunity* as the rest of the family but *not more*. This makes for a better-adjusted child *and* for better adjusted siblings.

As parents work with their child, they should keep a record of his progress. This will help them see the growth he has made. We have found the Speech and Language Development Table in Chapter I very helpful in charting progress. However, parents should not limit the record to speech growth. Changes should be noted in behavior, motor skills, attention span, initiation of play activities, and cooperation.

As stated before, the teacher has a number of advantages in working with a child other than the obvious one of better training for the task. This can easily lead parents into the attitude that they do not have the capabilities or background to help train their child. Nothing could be more in error or more tragic for the parent or the child. We must not lose sight of the fact that parents also have a number of advantages as educators which are usually denied to the teacher. Parents have a more flexible schedule which can be adapted to the constantly changing needs and varying length of attention and interest of the child. Also, parents may work in more familiar and hence more secure and relaxing surroundings. In addition, parents, of course, inspire much stronger feelings of love and desire to please than the teacher does.

It is important for parents to remember, as they work with the material in this book, that each child is an individual and no set program can fit the needs of all children. The parent-teacher must adapt the material in the preceding pages to fit the child's needs and must seek out the material suggested in the appendix and bibliography which is best for his child.

Training for the speech-delayed child cannot and should not be all drill and structured lessons. Language building and speech development go on all day long, and parents are the ones chiefly responsible for the earlier phases of stimulation and motivation.

They must talk, talk, talk to their child unremittingly, with infinite patience and without apparent concern or pressure for the child to use this speech productively.

Close behind stimulation would come motivation as a responsibility of the parents. The child must be convinced by the parents that speech is not an unpleasant, meaningless task to be performed as a parlor trick, but rather that speech is an extremely useful tool for gratifying his wants in the shortest time with a minimum expenditure of energy.

Moreover, by their behavior and attitude toward speech and the child's problems with it, parents must convince the child that communicating is a pleasant experience and that it is fun. Parents who constantly yell at each other and their children, or who bicker and "pick" verbally at each other, often give the young child the impression that speech is a very unpleasant thing and something for them to reject.

Finally, parents must learn to avoid dwelling on the long-range goals and milestones of progress and must look instead to the very small subgoals and footstones. This will bring not only reward and encouragement to the child in his speech efforts, but also real joy, sense of accomplishment, and encouragement to the parents as well. These times will make the frustrating moments worthwhile.

In conclusion, for a child to speak, he must have something to say, the need for saying it, security in the act of saying it; and sufficient praise, encouragement, and self-satisfaction to make the effort worthwhile.

Appendix I

Children's Books

For Speech and Language Stimulation

Albert Whitman and Co., Chicago:
  1. *A Button in Her Ear* by Ada B. Litchfield
  2. *Tell-A-Tale Series*
Crown Publishers, New York:
  1. *The Bear and the Fly* by Paula Winter
Dial Press, New York:
  1. *Why Mosquitos Buzz in People's Ears* by Verna Aardema
Dodd, Mead and Co., New York:
  1. *The Little Mother Goose* illustrated by Jessie Wilcox Smith
Doubleday, New York:
  1. *Red Light, Green Light* by Golden McDonald
E. P. Dutton and Co., New York:
  1. *Winnie the Pooh Stories* by A. A. Milne
Follett Publishing Co., New York:
  1. *Bendomelina* by Jan Slepian and Ann Seidler
  2. *The Hungry Thing* by Jan Slepian and Ann Seidler
Frederick Warne and Co., New York:
  1. *The Tale of Peter Rabbit* by Beatrix Potter
  2. *Ginger and Pickles* by Beatrix Potter
Golden Press, New York:
  1. Golden Books:
    The Three Bears
    The Shy Little Kitten
Grosset and Dunlap, New York:
  1. Wonder Books:
    Nonsense Alphabet
    Wonder Book of Trains
    Let's Go to School
  2. Wonder Starters:
    Airplanes
    Night

3. Big Books:
   Animals Every Child Should Know
   Book of Clowns

Harper and Row, New York:
1. *The Noisy Book* by Margaret Wise Brown
2. *All Falling Down* by Gene Zion
3. *The Duck* by Margaret Wise Brown
4. *Goodnight Moon* by Margaret Wise Brown
5. *The Storm Book* by Charlotte Zolotow
6. *The Tall Book of Nursery Tales* illustrated by Fiodor Rajankovsky

Henry Z. Walck, Inc., New York:
1. *Little Auto* by Lois Lenski
2. *Little Train and Little Airplane* by Lois Lenski
3. *Strawberry Girl* by Lois Lenski

J. B. Lippincott Co., Philadelphia:
1. *All Around the Town* by Phyllis McGinley

Pantheon Books, New York:
1. *Switch on the Night* by Ray Bradbury

Random House, New York:
1. Dr. Seuss Stories:
   Dr. Seuss ABC's
   The Cat in the Hat
   The Cat in the Hat Comes Back
   Hop on Pop
   Green Eggs and Ham
   Horton Hatches the Egg
   Horton Hears a Who
   McElligot's Pool
2. Beginning Reader Stories:
   Ten Apples Up On Top by Theodore LeSieg
   A Fish Out of Water by Helen Palmer
3. Babar Stories:
   Babar the King by Jean DeBrunhoff
   Babar and Zephir by Jean DeBrunhoff
4. Sesame Street Books:
   Sesame Street Muppets

5. Richard Scarry Books:
   ABC Wordbook
   Funniest Storybook Ever
   What Do People Do All Day

Simon and Schuster, New York:
   1. *Sylvester and the Magic Pebble* by William Steig

The Macmillan Co., New York:
   1. *The Box with Red Wheels* by Maud and Miska Petersham
   2. *One Fine Day* by Nonny Hogrogian

Thomas V. Cromwell, New York:
   1. *Read to Me Storybook* by The Child Study Association of America

Viking Press, New York:
   1. *Madeline* by Ludwig Bemelmans

Walker and Co., New York:
   1. *City ABC's* by Michael Deasy

William Morrow and Co., Inc., New York:
   1. *My Nursery School* by Harlow Rockwell

Young, Scott, Inc., New York:
   1. *A Child's Goodnight Book* by Margaret Wise Brown
   2. *While Suzie Sleeps* by Nina Schneider

CHILDREN'S MAGAZINES

Children's House
Children's House, Inc.
Post Office Box 111
Caldwell, N.J. 07006

Children Today
Superintendent of Documents
U.S. Government Printing Office
Washington, D.C.

Highlights for Children
2300 West 5th Avenue
Columbus, Ohio 43272

Humpty Dumpty's Magazine for Little Children
Parent's Magazine Enterprises, Inc.
Subscription Department
Bergenfield, N.J. 07621

Ranger Rick's Nature Magazine
National Wildlife Federation
1412 Sixteenth Street, N. W.
Washington, D.C. 20402

Sesame Street
Children's Television Workshop
Post Office Box C-10
Birmingham, Ala. 35201

Appendix II

Children's Records

For Speech and Language Stimulation

Due to the rapid changes in the publication and availability of children's records, it is difficult to compile an accurate listing of current record titles. Therefore, we have listed only a few examples of records best suited to stimulate the child with speech and language delay. Your public library or local record store may furnish you with additional suggestions.

Bowmar Records, Inc.:
   1. *Child's World of Sounds*

Children's Record Group:
   1. *The Carrot Seed*
   2. *Me, Myself and I*
   3. *Train to the Zoo*

Children's Records of America:
   1. Sesame Street Record Series:
     Ernie's Hits
     Electric Company

Disneyland Records:
   1. *Emperor's New Clothes*
   2. *Walt Disney Fun with Music*
   3. *Winnie the Pooh*
   4. *A Little Golden Book and Record*

Peter Pan:
   1. *Let's Play the New Romper Room Games*

Vocalion:
   1. *Babar Songs and Stories*
   2. *Child's First Record Series*

Appendix III

Parent's Books

For Speech and Language Stimulation

1. Brazelton, T. Berry, M.D.: Toddlers and Parents, *A Declaration of Independence.* Delacorte Pr, Semour Lawrence, 1974.
2. Collins, Norman et al.: *Teach Your Child to Talk, A Parent Handbook.* New York, CEBCO/Standard Pub, 1975.
3. Editor: *Correspondence Course for Parents of Preschool Deaf and Hard-of-Hearing Children.* Los Angeles, John Tracy Clinic, 806 Adams Blvd., Los Angeles, California.
4. Lehane, Stephen: *Help Your Baby Learn.* Englewood Cliffs, P-H, 1976.
5. Lowell, Edgar and Stoner, Marguerite: *Play It by Ear, Auditory Training Games.* Los Angeles, John Tracy Clinic, 1963.
6. National Institute of Health: *Learning to Talk; Speech, Hearing and Language Problems in the Pre-School Child.* Washington, U.S. Government Printing Office, 1975.
7. Painter, Genevieve: *Teach Your Baby.* New York, S&S, 1971.

Appendix IV

ORGANIZATIONS which are interested in the Speech, Language, and Hearing Handicapped Child:

VOLUNTARY AND PROFESSIONAL ORGANIZATIONS

1. American Association on Mental Deficiency, Inc., 5201 Connecticut Avenue, N.W., Washington, D.C. 20015
2. American Association of Psychiatric Clinics for Children, 250 West 57th Street, New York, N.Y. 10019
3. American Montessori Society, 175 Fifth Avenue, New York, N.Y. 10010
4. American Speech and Hearing Association, 10801 Rockville Pike, Rockville, MD 20852
5. American Psychological Association, Inc., 1200 Seventeenth Street, N.W., Washington, D.C. 20036
6. Association for Children with Learning Disabilities, 2200 Brownsville Road, Pittsburgh, PA 15201
7. Better Hearing Institute, 1001 Connecticut Avenue, N.W., Suite 632, Washington, D.C. 20036
8. Child Welfare League of America, Inc., 67 Irving Place, New York, N.Y. 10003
9. Council for Exceptional Children, 1411 South Jefferson Davis Highway, Suite 900, Arlington, VA 22202
10. National Association for Autistic Children, 621 Central Avenue, Albany, N.Y. 12206
11. National Association for Mental Health, Inc., 1800 North Kent Street, Rosslyn, Arlington, VA 22209
12. National Association for Retarded Children, 2705 Avenue "E" East, Arlington, TX 76011
13. National Association of Hearing and Speech Action, 814 Thayer Avenue, Silver Spring, MD 20910
14. National Society for Crippled Children and Adults, 2023 West Ogden, Chicago, IL 60612
15. The Alexander Graham Bell Association for the Deaf, 3417 Volta Place, N.W., Washington, D.C. 20007
16. United Cerebral Palsy Association, Inc., 66 East 34th Street, New York, N.Y. 10016

Appendix V

Directories for Professional Workers and Schools for Speech, Language, and Hearing

Annual Directory
American Speech and Hearing Association
10801 Rockville Pike
Rockville, MD 20852

Directory of Services for the Deaf in the United States
American Annals of the Deaf
Gallaudet College
Washington, D.C. 20002

Guide to Clinical Services in Speech Pathology and Audiology
10801 Rockville Pike
Rockville, MD 20852

International Directory of Schools and Organizations for the Deaf
American Annals of the Deaf
Gallaudet College
Washington, D.C. 20002

National Register of Health Service Providers in Psychology
1200 Seventeenth Street, N.W.
Washington, D.C. 20036

JOURNALS OR PUBLICATIONS

Closer Look
Special Education Information Center
1828 L Street, N.W.
Washington, D.C. 20036

Hearing and Speech Action
National Association for Hearing and Speech Action
814 Thayer Avenue
Silver Spring, MD 20910

Hearing News
American Hearing Society
817 Fourteenth Street, N.W.
Washington, D.C.

Information Office
National Institute of Neurological Diseases and Stroke
National Institute of Health
United States Department of Health, Education and Welfare
Bethesda, MD 20014

The Exceptional Parent
Post Office Box 4944
Manchester, NH 03108

Volta Review
The Alexander Graham Bell Association for the Deaf
3417 Volta Place, N.W.
Washington, D.C. 20007

Bibliography

ARTICLES

Battin, R. Ray: The development of language. *International Child Welfare Review*, No. 13, April, 1972.

Battin R. Ray and Kraft, Irvin A.: Psycholinguistic evaluation of children referred for private consultation to a child psychiatrist. *Journal of Learning Disabilities*, Vol. I, pp. 600-605, 1968.

Baumrind, Diana: Parental control and parental love. *Children, 12*:230-234, 1965.

Downs, Marion P.: Hearing loss, definition, epidemiology and prevention. *Public Health Review*, Vol. IV. July-Dec, pp. 225-380, 1975.

Downs, Marion P.: The establishment of hearing aid use; a program for parents. Maico Audiological Library Series. Vol. IV, 1967.

DuBois, F. S.: The security of discipline. *Ment Hyg, 36*:353-372, 1952.

Haug, Olaf, Baccaro, Paul and Guilford, Frederick R.: A pure-tone audiogram on the infant, the PIWI technique. *Archives of Otolaryngology*, 86:435-440, 1967.

Kraft, I. and Battin, R. Ray: The under achiever. *Journal of the American Medical Women's Association*, July, pp. 343-348, 1973.

Lewis, Neil: Otitis media and linguistic incompetence. *Archives of Otolaryngology*, Vol. 102, July, pp. 387-390, 1976.

Noshpitz, Joseph D.: Can you say "no" to your child? *Children's House*, Nov-Dec, pp. 6-9, 1966.

Sheer, D. E.: Is there a common factor in learning for brain injured children? *Except Child, 21*:10-12, 1954.

BOOKS

Abney, Louise and Miniaco, Dorothy: *This Way to Better Speech.* Yonkers-on-Hudson, N. Y., World Book Co. 1940.

Anderson, Virgil A.: *Improving the Child's Speech.* New York, Oxford U. Pr, 1954.

Beasley, Jane: *Slow to Talk; A Guide for Teachers and Parents of Children with Delayed Language Development.* New York, Bureau of Publications, Teachers College, Columbia University, 1959.

Biebe, H. H.: *A Guide to Help the Severely Hard of Hearing Child.* New York, Karger, S., 1953.

Birch, Jack W., Matthews, Jack and Burgi, Ernest: *Improving Children's Speech.* Cincinnati, Public School Publishing Company, 1958.

Bibliography

Collins, Norman et al.: *Teach Your Child to Talk, A Parent Handbook.* New York, CEBCO/Standard Publishing, 1975.
Dunn, Lloyd M. and Smith, James O.: *Peabody Language Development Kits.* Minnesota, American Guidance Service, Inc., 1966.
Downs, Marion P.: Deafness in Childhood. In Best, Fred (Ed.): *The International Symposium on Deafness in Children.* June, 1976.
Editor: *Correspondence Course for Parents of Preschool Deaf and Hard-of-Hearing Children.* Los Angeles, John Tracy Clinic, 806 Adams Blvd., Los Angeles, California.
Faber, Adele and Mazlish, Elaine: *Liberated Parents, Liberated Children.* New York, Grosset and Dunlap, 1974.
Flavell, John H.: *The Developmental Psychology of Jean Piaget.* New York, Van Nostrand Reinhold Co., 1963.
Gesell, A. et al.: *The First Five Years of Life.* New York, Harper, 1940.
Gesell, Arnold et al.: *Infant and Child in the Culture of Today; The Guidance of Development in Home and Nursery School.* New York, Harper, 1943.
Ginott, Haim G.: *Betwen Parent and Child.* New York, Macmillan, 1965.
Hodgson, W. R.: Testing Infants and Young Children. In Katz, J. (Ed.): *Handbook of Clinical Audiology.* Baltimore, Williams and Wilkins, 1972.
Johnson, Wendell: *Speech Problems of Children.* New York, Grune, 1950.
Keiser, Armilda B.: *Here's How and Why.* New York, Friendship, 1953.
Kratoville, Betty Lou and Schweich, Peter (Eds.): *Hyperactivity: A Meeting of the Minds.* New York, Parent Press, 1977.
Lassman, Grace: *Language for the Preschool Deaf Child.* New York, Grune, 1950.
Lenneberg, E. H.: The natural history of language. In Smith, F. and Miller, G. (Eds.): *The Genesis of Language.* Cambridge, The M.I.T. Press, 1966.
Lenneberg, E. H.: *Biological Foundation of Language.* New York, Wiley, 1967.
Lewis, M. M.: *How Children Learn to Speak.* London, George G. Harrap and Co. Ltd., 1957.
Lewis, R., Strauss, A. and Lehtinen, L.: *The Other Child.* New York, Grune, 1960.
Lowell, E. L. and Stoner, M.: *Play It by Ear,* Los Angeles, John Tracy Clinic, 1960.
McCarthy, D.: Language development in children. In Carmichael, L. (Ed.): *Manual of Child Psychology,* 2nd ed. New York, Wiley, 1954.
McCarthy, D.: *The Language Development of the Preschool Child.* (Institute of Child Welfare Monographs, Sec. No. 4). Minneapolis, U of Minn Pr, 1930.
Meier, John H.: Learning disabilities found in the schools. In Satz, Paul

and Ross, John L. (Eds.): *The Disabled Learner.* Groningen, Rotterdam U Pr, 1972.

Miller, M. H. and Polisar, I. A.: *Audiological Evaluation of the Pediatric Patient.* Springfield. Thomas, 2nd Printing, 1971.

Morkovin, Boris and Moore, Lucilia M.: *Through the Barriers of Deafness and Isolation.* New York, 1960.

Myklebust, Helmer: *Auditory Disorders in Children.* New York, Grune, 1954.

Myklebust, Helmer: *Your Deaf Child.* Springfield, Thomas, 1950.

Northern, Jerry L. and Downs, Marion P.: *Hearing in Children.* Baltimore, Williams & Wilkins, 1974.

Painter, Genevieve: *Teach Your Baby.* New York, S&S, 1971.

Palmer, Charles E.: *Speech and Hearing Problems.* Springfield, Thomas, 1961.

Pollack, D.: *Educational Audiology for the Limited Hearing Infant.* Springfield, Thomas, 1970.

Schoolfield, Lucille D.: *Better Speech and Better Reading.* Boston, Expression, 1951.

Scott, Louise Binder and Thompson, J. J.: *Talking Time for Speech Correction and Speech Improvement.* St. Louis, Webster Pub. Co., 1951.

Silverman, S. R. and Lane, H. S.: Deaf Children. In Davis, H. and Silverman, S. R. (Eds.): *Hearing and Deafness,* 3rd ed. New York, H.R.&W., 1970.

Stinchfield, Hawk Sara: The learning and development of speech; learning to speak effectively. *Bulletin of the Association for Childhood Education,* 1944, pp. 9-10.

Thompson, Evelyn S.: *A Handbook for Phonetic and Structural Analysis in Reading.* Houston, College of Education, University of Houston, 1957.

Tracy, Richmond et al.: *If You Have a Deaf Child.* Urbana, U of Ill Pr, 1959.

Utley, Jean: *What's Its Name.* Urbana, U of Ill Pr, 1950. (Auditory Training Album Optional.)

Van Riper, Charles: The importance of speech; learning to speak effectively. *Bulletin of the Association for Childhood Education.* Washington, 1944.

Van Riper, Charles: *Teaching Your Child to Talk.* New York, Harper, 1950.

Webber, Robert E.: Early Childhood Development. In Webber, Robert E. (Ed.): *Handbook on Learning Disabilities.* Englewood Cliffs, P-H, Inc., 1974.

Whitehurst, M. W.: *Auditory Training for Children.* New York, Hearing Rehabilitation Center, 1949.

PAMPHLETS

Chapin, Amy B. and Corcoran, Margaret: *A Child Doesn't Talk.* Cleveland Jr. Chamber of Commerce, 400 Union Commerce Bldg., Cleveland, Ohio.
Better Living Booklets: Science Research Associates, Inc., 57 W. Grand Avenue, Chicago 10, Illinois.
Foster, Constance J.: *Developing Responsibility in Children.* 1953.
Grossman, Jean Sebick and LeShan, Eda J.: *How Children Play—for Fun and Learning.* 1951.
Krug, Othelda I. and Beck, Helen L.: *A Guide to Better Discipline.* 1954.
Olsen, Willard C. and Lewellen, John: *How Children Grow and Develop.* 1953.
Ridenour, Nina: *Building Self-Confidence in Children.* 1951.
Van Riper, Charles: *Helping Children to Talk Better.* 1951.
Consumer's Guide: *Facts about Hearing and Hearing Aids.* Washington, National Bureau of Standards. U. S. Department of Commerce.
Long, Paul E.: *Teaching with the Flannelboard.* Philadelphia, Jacronda Mfg. Co., 1957.
Moffat, S.: *Helping the Child Who Cannot Hear.* New York. The Public Affairs Committee, Public Affairs Pamphlet No. 479, 1972.
Wood, Nancy: *Language Disorders in Children.* Chicago, National Society for Crippled Children and Adults, Inc., 1959.

Author Index

A
Abney, L., 92
Anderson, V. A., 23, 92

B
Baccaro, P., 76, 92
Battin, R. R., 11, 58, 79, 92
Baumrind, D., 19, 92
Beasley, J., 92
Beck, H. L., 19, 95
Biebe, H. H., 75, 92
Birch, J. W., 92
Brazelton, T., 88
Burgi, E., 92

C
Chapin, A. B., 95
Collins, N., 39, 88, 93
Corcoran, M., 95

D
Downs, M. P., 24, 39, 75, 76, 92, 93, 94
DuBois, F. S., 19, 92
Dunn, L. M., 93

E
Eisenson, J., 58

F
Faber, A., 19, 93
Flavell, J. H., 79, 93
Foster, C. J., 19, 95

G
Gesell, A., 11, 93
Ginott, H. G., 17, 19, 93
Grossman, J. S., 95
Guilford, F. R., 76, 92

H
Haug, O., 76, 92
Hodgson, W. R., 76, 93

J
Johnson, K. O., 11
Johnson, W., 93

K
Keiser, A. B., 93
Kraft, I. A., 58, 79, 92
Kratoville, B. L., 19, 93
Krug, O. I., 19, 95

L
Lane, H. S., 76, 94
Lassman, G., 76, 93
Lehane, S., 88
Lehtinen, L., 93
Lenneberg, E. H., 3, 11, 12, 93
LeShan, E. J., 95
Lewellen, J., 12, 95
Lewis, M. M., 12, 93
Lewis, N., 39, 92, 93
Long, P. E., 95
Lowell, E. L., 85, 93

M
Matthews, J., 92
Mazlish, E., 19, 93
McCarthy, D., 12, 93
Meier, J. H., 79, 93
Miller, M. H., 76, 94
Miniaco, D., 92
Moffat, S., 76, 95
Moore, L. M., 94
Morkovin, B., 94
Myklebust, H., 23, 76, 94

N
Northern, J. L., 39, 76, 94
Noshpitz, J. D., 19, 92

O
Olsen, W. C., 12, 95

P

Painter, G., 88, 94
Palmer, C. E., 94
Piaget, J., 77
Polisar, I. A., 76, 94
Pollack, D., 76, 94

R

Ridenour, N., 95
Ronnei, E., 76

S

Schoolfield, L. D., 94
Schweich, P., 19, 93
Scott, L. B., 94
Sheer, D. E., 42, 92
Silverman, S. R., 76, 94
Smith, J. O., 93
Stinchfield, H. S., 94
Stoner, M., 88, 93
Strauss, A., 93

T

Thompson, E. S., 94
Thompson, J. J., 94
Tracy, R., 76, 94

U

Utley, J., 76, 94

V

Van Riper, C., 42, 94, 95

W

Webber, R. E., 79, 94
Whitehurst, M. W., 94
Wood, N. E., 13, 23, 95

Subject Index

A

ABC Wordbook, 85
A Button in Her Ear, 83
Acceptance, 11
Adjectives, 78
Adverbs, 78
Airplanes, 83
Alexander Graham Bell Association for the Deaf, 89
All Around the Town, 84
All Falling Down, 84
American Association of Psychiatric Clinics for Children, 89
American Association on Mental Deficiency, Inc., 89
American Psychological Association, Inc., 89
American Speech and Hearing Association, viii, 11, 89
 annual directory, 90
Animals Every Child Should Know, 84
Articulation development, 78
Articulation training, 23
Association for Children with Learning Disabilities, 89
Attention, 13
Attention span, 8, 20, 55, 78, 81
Auditory abnormalities, 24
Auditory perception, 47, 52-57
 closure, 52
 discrimination, 70-72
 memory, increasing, 8, 53-55
 recall, immediate, 52
 retention, long-term, 52
  increasing, 53-55
 selective attention, 52
 sequential memory, 52
 sound blending, 52
Autonomy, 18-19

B

Babar and Zephir, 84
Babar Songs and Stories, 87
Babar the King, 84
Babbling, 4, 43
Baby talk, 22
Basic skills, maturation of, 77
Bead chain, 60
Bear and the Fly, The, 83
Behavior changes, 81
Behavior deviations, 13
Behavior problems, 58
Bendomelina, 83
Better Hearing Institute, 89
Bilabial sounds, 43, 47
Blocks, building, 60
Book of Clowns, 84
Books
 children's, 83-85
 parent's, 88
 reading, 28
Box With Red Wheels, The, 85
Brain injury, 13
 freedom from, 8
Brain Stem Evoked Response, 69
Bribes, 17

C

Carrot Seed, The, 87
Cat in the Hat, The, 84
Cat in the Hat Comes Back, The, 84
Child Welfare League of America, Inc., 89
Children Today, 85
Children's House, 85
Child's First Record Series, 87
Child's Goodnight Book, A, 85
Child's World of Sounds, 87
Chronic illness, freedom from, 8
City ABC's, 85
Clay, modeling, 34
Closer Look, 90
Colors, 78
Comparatives, 78
Confidence, 18
Consistency, 17

Consonants, 47
Cooperation, 81
Correspondence Course for Parents of Preschool Deaf and Hard-of-Hearing Children, 88
Council for Exceptional Children, 89
Counting, 79

D

Declaration of Independence, A, 88
Directions, understanding, 78
Directory of Services for the Deaf in the United States, 90
Discipline, 11
  speech and language, role in, 13-19
Distractibility, 13
Dollhouse, 33
Do's and don'ts, 15
Dot to dot designs, 63
Dr. Seuss ABC's, 84
Drawing, 64
Duck, The, 84

E

Ear training, 20, 43-51
  methods for initiating, 43-51
Echolalia, 5, 7, 43, 45
Electric Company, 22, 87
Electric Response Audiometry, 69
Electro-cochleography, 69
Emotional balance, 8
Emperor's New Clothes, 87
Environmental sounds, 43
Ernie's Hits, 87
Example, being an, 18
Exceptional Parent, The, 91
Eye movements, 79

F

Facial expression, 42
Fish Out of Water, A, 84
Flannel board, 29, 50, 62
Follow the Leader, 55
Form perception, 31, 32, 33
Funniest Storybook Ever, 85

G

Gestures, 40
Ginger and Pickles, 83

Goodnight Moon, 84
Green Eggs and Ham, 84
Gross-sound drill, 45
Guide to Clinical Services in Speech Pathology and Audiology, 90

H

Hard-of-hearing child, 65-75
Hearing aid, 69, 70
  binaural, 7
  care, 72-74
  ear placement, 74-75
  types, 71
  wearing adjustments, 75
Hearing and Speech Action, 90
Hearing loss, 24, 52, 58
  sensorineural, 25, 26
Hearing News, 91
Hearing, normal, 8, 24
Hearing testing, 25, 65
  puppet in window illuminated technique, 66-69
Help Your Baby Learn, 88
Highlights, 64, 85
Hop on Pop, 84
Horton Hatches the Egg, 84
Horton Hears a Who, 84
Humpty Dumpty's Magazine for Little Children, 85
Hungry Thing, The, 83

I

Imagery, poor verbal, 52
Imitation, 7
Individuality, 19
Instruction, verbal, 16
Intelligence, adequate, 8
International Directory of Schools and Organizations for the Deaf, 90
Intrafamily relationships, healthy, 11

K

Kinesthetic cues, 34

L

Lallation, 5, 7, 43
Language building program
  auditory and visual memory, 20

Subject Index

ear training, 20
motivation, 20
stimulation, 20
Language, definition of, 3
Language development, 3-11, 9-10 (table)
  auditory perception, 52-57
  basic requirements, 8, 11
  don'ts, 22-23
  do's, 21-22
  ear training, 43-51
  visual perception, 58-64
Language retarded therapy program, 20-23
Learning difficulties, 59
Learning to Talk, 88
Legos, 38
Let's Go to School, 83
Let's Play the New Romper Room Games, 87
Likenesses and differences, recognizing, 79
Limits, security of, 14
Lipreading skills, 58, 70-72
Listening activities, advanced, 56-57
Listening exercises, 45
Listening habits, 45
Lite Brite, 38
Little Auto, 84
Little Golden Book and Record, 87
Little Mother Goose, The, 83
Little Train and Little Airplane, 84
Lotto games, 28
Love, 18

M

Madeline, 85
Magazines, children's, 85-86
Mastoid bone conduction, 69
Matching objects, 62
McElligot's Pool, 84
Me, Myself and I, 87
Middle ear disease, 25, 26
Motor skills, 81
My Nursery School, 85

N

National Association for Autistic Children, 89
National Association for Mental Health, Inc., 89
National Association for Retarded Children, 89
National Association of Hearing and Speech Action, 89
National Institute of Neurological Disease and Stroke, 91
National Register of Health Service Providers in Psychology, 90
National Society for Crippled Children and Adults, 89
Night, 83
Noise imitation, 38
Noisemakers, 53
Noisy Book, The, 84
Nonsense Alphabet, 83

O

One Fine Day, 85
Opposites, common, 78
Organization, voluntary and professional, 89

P

Painting, 35-37
Parent as teacher, 80-82
Patience, parental, 20
Pediacoumeter, vi
Pegboard, 38, 60
Perfection, avoiding, 18
Perseveration, 13
Picture cards, matching, 28, 53
Play It by Ear, Auditory Training Games, 88
Praise, 17
Prepositions, 78
Pretend play, 39
Promises, verbal, 22
Punishment, 14, 17-18
Puppets, hand, 33
Puzzles, simple, 28, 60

R

Ranger Rick's Nature Magazine, 86
Read to Me Storybook, 85
Reasonability, 15
Records, children's, 87

Red Light, Green Light, 83
Repetition, 27
Rhythm exercises, 45
Rhythm, sense of, 38
Routine, establishing, 13, 14-15
Rules, 14-15

S

School readiness, 77-79
Security, 11
Self-control, 13
Self-discipline, 78
Sensitivity Prediction from Acoustic Reflex, 69
Sensory deprivation, 24
Sentence length, 78
Serial-number stimulation, 38
Serous otitis media, 24
Sesame Street, 22
Sesame Street magazine, 86
Sesame Street Muppets, 84
Shy Little Kitten, The, 83
Simon Says, 45, 55
Sitting time, 55
Socialization, 78
Sorting objects, 62
Sound discrimination, 44
Spatial orientation, 79
Spatial relations, 27
Speech
  definition, 3
  development, 3-11, 9-10 (table)
    basic requirements, 8, 11
    don'ts, 22-23
    do's, 21-22
    motivation, 40-42
  disorders, 11
  parts of, 27
  sound combinations, 47
    reception and understanding, 44
  standards, good, 11
  true, 7
Speech-handicapped, stimulation of, 24-39
Stimulation, language, 11, 24-39
  home, in, 26-39
Stories, making up, 29-31

Storm Book, The, 84
Strawberry Girl, 84
Switch on the Night, 84
Sylvester and the Magic Pebble, 85

T

Tale of Peter Rabbit, The, 83
Tall Book of Nursery Tales, The, 84
Teach Your Baby, 88
Teach Your Child to Talk, 88
Tell-A-Tale Series, 83
Temper tantrums, 13, 41
Ten Apples Up on Top, 84
Threats, verbal, 22
Three Bears, The, 83
Tinker Toys, 38
Tongue tips, 47
Train to the Zoo, 87
Trust, 18
"Tuning in," 15-16

U

United Cerebral Palsy Association, Inc., 89

V

Verb tenses, 78
Visual perception, 58-64
  closure, 58
  discrimination, 58
  memory, 58
  sequencing, 58
Visual training, 59-64
  supplies, 59
Vocabulary size, 78
Volta Review, 91
Vowels, 47

W

Walt Disney Fun With Music, 87
What Do People Do All Day, 85
While Suzie Sleeps, 85
Why Mosquitos Buzz in People's Ears, 83
Winnie the Pooh, 87
Winnie the Pooh Stories, 83
Wonder Book of Trains, 83